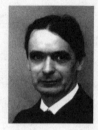

RUDOLF STEINER (1861–1925) called
his spiritual philosophy 'anthroposophy',
meaning 'wisdom of the human being'. As a
highly developed seer, he based his work on
direct knowledge and perception of spiritual
dimensions. He initiated a modern and
universal 'science of spirit', accessible to
anyone willing to exercise clear and unprejudiced thinking.

From his spiritual investigations Steiner provided sugges-
tions for the renewal of many activities, including education
(both general and special), agriculture, medicine, econ-
omics, architecture, science, philosophy, religion and the
arts. Today there are thousands of schools, clinics, farms and
other organizations involved in practical work based on his
principles. His many published works feature his research
into the spiritual nature of the human being, the evolution of
the world and humanity, and methods of personal development. Steiner wrote some 30 books and delivered over 6000
lectures across Europe. In 1924 he founded the General
Anthroposophical Society, which today has branches
throughout the world.

EURYTHMY THERAPY

*Eight Lectures given in Dornach, Switzerland, between
12 and 18 April 1921 and in Stuttgart, Germany, on
28 October 1922*

RUDOLF STEINER

RUDOLF STEINER PRESS

Translated by Alan Stott

Rudolf Steiner Press
Hillside House, The Square
Forest Row, RH18 5ES

www.rudolfsteinerpress.com

Second edition published by Rudolf Steiner Press 2009

Previously published in an earlier translation under the title *Curative Eurythmy* by Rudolf Steiner Press in 1983

Originally published in German under the title *Heileurythmie* (volume 315 in the *Rudolf Steiner Gesamtausgabe* or Collected Works) by Rudolf Steiner Verlag, Dornach. This authorized translation, based on the fifth edition, is published by permission of the Rudolf Steiner Nachlassverwaltung, Dornach

A catalogue record for this book is available from the British Library

ISBN: 978 1 85584 224 3

Cover by Andrew Morgan; cover photo by John Playfoot
Typeset by DP Photosetting, Neath, West Glamorgan
Printed and bound in Malta by Gutenberg Press Ltd.

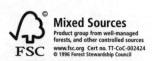

Mixed Sources
Product group from well-managed forests, and other controlled sources
www.fsc.org Cert no. TT-CoC-002424
© 1996 Forest Stewardship Council

The paper used for this book is FSC-certified and totally chlorine-free. FSC (the Forest Stewardship Council) is an international network to promote responsible management of the world's forests.

Contents

Synopsis of the Lectures

Lecture 1
Dornach, 12 April 1921, p.m.
The relationship of the health-stimulating, therapeutic element of eurythmy to the educational and artistic element of eurythmy. The larynx and metamorphosis. The larynx as an etheric, second human being within man. The frontal lobe and the thyroid. The eurythmy carried out by the larynx in speaking and singing. Stasis of the head and dynamics of the rhythmic system; rhythm and a-rhythm and their connections with thinking. The actual effect on the human being of logic, syntax and prose, and rhythm and poetry. The falling apart of the coherence of a system striving forwards and backwards. Iambic and trochaic exercises. The connection between movement of the limbs and the manner of thinking. Digestion and headaches. Writing with the feet. 'I-A-O' exercises. What is felt in the limbs as the essential element of eurythmical movement. The primal A (*eh*) in the crossing of the axes of vision. Eurythmy in groups for health and therapy. Form of the organs and movement-forms.

Lecture 2
Dornach, 13 April 1921, p.m.
The character of vowels and consonants. Speech and movement in close connection in earlier times; this becomes looser in our time. Bringing the body into movement again in eurythmy. Bringing the various eurythmical vowels into the realm of therapy: 'I', 'U', 'O', 'E', 'A'. The arm movements and indications for the individual vowels and doing vowels in

general. Leg movements to the vowel exercises. Inner photography as the effective therapeutic element in doing consonants. 'M', 'S', 'H' in relationship to Lucifer and Ahriman.

Lecture 3
Dornach, 14 April 1921, p.m.
The coming-to-grips with the outer world in the consonantal element in speech; in speaking vowels, the coming to oneself through an inner activity. The three principles at work in the consonants and their effect. The vowels tingeing the sounds of speech; movement as the polar opposite to actual speaking—blowing sounds, plosives, vibrating and wave sounds; lip, teeth and palate sounds and the mutual alternation of the differentiating principle. The physiological processes in speaking the vowels 'A', 'U', 'O', 'E' and their polar effect in eurythmy therapy. Movement in the will and movement in the intellect. The losing of the formative quality of language by the intellect as the inner cause of illness. Becoming ill through civilization and the stimulation to health of eurythmy.

Lecture 4
Dornach, 15 April 1921, p.m.
Vowels work directly upon the rhythmic organism; the consonants work upon it via the organism of the metabolism and limbs. The eurythmical therapeutic metamorphosis of the movement of the consonants: 'B/P', 'D/T', 'G/K/Q', 'S', 'F', 'R', 'L', 'H', 'M', 'N', 'Sh' and their effects. Connections between the system of movement and the digestive system. Eurythmy as ensouled gymnastics. Speaking vowels before the eurythmy therapy vowel exercise. Afterwards, listening

with the soul and spirit to what has moved. Bringing life and movement into the human etheric body. The 'R'-movement and its use in education. Regulating an over-strong effect in therapy.

Lecture 5
Dornach, 16 April 1921, p.m.
Twelve eurythmical exercises to work from the soul element into the whole constitution of the organism via the etheric body—judgement; expression of will; movement of feeling— 'E'; movement of wish—'U'; movement of bending and stretching with 'B', 'R', 'M'; dexterity—'E'; 'E' and 'O' as forms to move in space; 'H-A' and 'A-H'. Making the etheric body supple. The application of these exercises in education, eurythmy for health and therapy. Physiological gymnastics as the school of materialism; the effect of eurythmical gymnastics for human self-knowledge and self-control. Some questions regarding special cases answered. Advice to alternate the exercises and how long they should be kept up.

Lecture 6
Dornach, 17 April 1921, p.m.
The initial, spiritually orientated physiological element of eurythmy, with the example of Goethe's poem *Über allen Gipfeln ist Ruh*. Active listening is a condition akin to sleep, similar to Imagining. The ether-movements of the person who is asleep or who, while awake, is listening, are made visible by the physical body in carrying out eurythmy. Stimulation of the forces of growth in children; rejuvenating forces in adults. Effect of doing the vowels on the organs of the rhythmic system. Listening to the consonants. Effect of carrying out the consonants in eurythmy on the head-

organization. The process of digestion as the activity of transforming matter which unfolds towards the rhythmic system. Activity of the human will. The forces of egoism in their significance for the human organism. The forces of crystallization and the sculpting, plastic forces of the organs. Spiritual activity and physical activity. Rhythmic alternation of doing consonants and vowels in eurythmy. The effect on the human aura.

Lecture 7
Dornach, 18 April 1921, p.m. (held for physicians and medical students)
The forming of the earth and the formation of metals. The formative forces raying in from the cosmos concentrate around a centre through the forces of consolidation. The pushing forces of magnesium; the rounding forces of fluorine. The process of secretion as the mediating element between the formative forces and the forces of consolidation. The process of perception as a continuation of the process of becoming (formative forces—secretion—consolidation) and its reversal in ascending to Imagination, Inspiration and Intuition. The unconscious forces of Imagination called up through consonantal movements; case examples. Normalizing effect of doing the vowels in eurythmy on deformities of the rhythmic system. The shining process of the kidneys and occult drawings. Mechthild von Magdeburg. Doing beautiful poems in eurythmy, the effect on congenital illness. Changes in the breathing rhythm through doing the vowels in eurythmy; the breathing exercises of yoga. Penetrating power of conviction in relation to mainstream medicine. Dismissal of quacks within the anthroposophical movement.

Lecture 8

Stuttgart, 28 October 1922 (during the 'medical week' for physicians and medical students)

The meaning and significance of eurythmy therapy. The collaboration in human speech of the system of digestion and the system of the nerves and the senses. Eurythmy as the metamorphosis of the usual language of speech sounds through strengthening the will-nature and weakening the life of mental images. The general healthy effect of eurythmy therapy. Reflecting within of the eurythmical forming of eurythmy therapy through repetition. The practice of eurythmy therapy through a physician or the inner agreement with the physician. Healthy diagnosis. The working together of the vowel and consonantal elements with the example of teeth, 'L', 'A', 'O'; with the example of kidney infection, 'S', 'A', 'B', 'P'. The human organs observed in the polarity of centrifugal and centripetal dynamics; mutual regulation through eurythmy therapy. Sensitivity and an artistic disposition. Eurythmy therapy and established therapy. Massage. Gymnastics. 'E'-movement for strengthening; 'I'-movement to associate the right and left sides of the organism, with index finger and large toe, with the eyes. The complete 'U'-form in eurythmy therapy, standing to attention. 'O'-form, feeling the entire muscular system. Consciousness as a factor in the healing process. 'E'-forms and 'U'-forms regulate the connecting activities of the astral and etheric organism. Gentle eurythmy therapy with pregnant women; gynaecological problems; abdominal complaints. A warning against overrating the method; dilettantism. A healthy physiology as the basis for a therapy working in the light of day. Meeting misunderstandings.

Notes on the Translation

This is a new translation of eight lectures on eurythmy therapy, seven of which were held in Dornach during the afternoons of 12–18 April 1921, and one in Stuttgart, 28 October 1922. These lectures are included in the Catalogue of Rudolf Steiner's Complete Works as No. 315 (GA 315), previously published in an English translation by Kristina Krohn under the title *Curative Eurythmy*, London, Rudolf Steiner Press, 1983. The previous translation has also been consulted in making the present translation.

The German text used in the present translation is the 5th edition (Dornach 2003), which is published together with the therapy lectures for doctors given on the same days during the mornings (GA 313) (5th ed. Dornach 2001). Both these lecture courses, GA 313 and GA 315, are also available in the paperback series No. 755 (ISBN 3-7274-7550-1). The 16 lectures are published in chronological order. This thoroughly checked and revised German edition includes a note to the new edition written by Walter Kugler of the Rudolf Steiner Nachlassverwaltung, Dornach, which is responsible for Steiner's literary estate. Dr Kugler revised and enlarged the section of notes which form the basis of those in the present edition.

Some linguistic points of the present translation

This translation attempts accurately to render the lecturer's meaning in contemporary English as used in Britain. The earlier, more literal translation of *Heileurythmie*, 'curative eurythmy', was changed to 'eurythmy therapy' over 25 years ago by members of the profession in Britain, since eurythmists technically do not claim to 'heal' but to offer therapy. The current term in America is 'therapeutic eurythmy'. Again, *hygienisch*, 'hygienic', could suggest unsavoury associations in English. As a rule, this translation avoids the term, as it does the word 'cleansing'; for *hygienische Eurythmie* the phrase 'eurythmy for health' is employed as a workable alternative. *Methodisch-didakfisch* is a customary term relating to educational methods and instruction, and these English terms are the ones used here. Again, 'pedagogy' (from the Greek), a normal term for American and other English-users who have closer historical links to the German language, is in English a formal term for the more widespread term 'education'. 'Pedagogy' and 'pedagogical' is used more in moral contexts—a pedagogical event or course does you good, perhaps teaching patience and similar things. To English ears 'pedagogical', sounding so close to 'pedantic', has fallen out of general use today.

'Eurythmic', the adjective, is as innocent as, say, 'gymnastic', but since a well-known pop group has made its mark in general consciousness, the suggestion has been taken up here to spell the adjective 'eurythmical' in the attempt to avoid any irrelevant associations.

In this translation, for *das Ich* both of the following are used—'the "I" ' (with the inverted commas, since the first-person pronoun is not usually a noun) and the Latin word 'the ego' (used by many earlier translators). Needless to say, the latter is not used here with the meaning it has in some schools of psychology. Yet this word, 'the ego', is sometimes chosen here, especially in order to avoid any confusion when the vowel 'I' (*ee*) enters the discussion. Imagination, Inspiration and Intuition, as three technical terms in spiritual science, are distinguished with a capital letter.

For *plastisch*, the equivalent word is 'plastic', meaning 'sculptural, modelled'. Despite the influence of industrial overproduction on our language, the word 'plastic' is nevertheless retained here, especially in Lecture 7 where it is used in the interests of accuracy. However, 'sculptural' has also been used in this translation. In Lecture 7 *Absonderung* ('separating') is translated as 'secretion', *Aussonderung* ('expelling') as 'excretion', *Krafte des Befestigens* is rendered 'forces of consolidation' but could also be translated as 'forces of binding or anchoring'.

In the interests of accuracy of translation, as opposed to the pedantries of transliteration (abhorred by Steiner himself) the editor has reduced the 'musts' of Steiner's perfectly polite German, employed more participles as natural for English, broken up occasional over-long sentences into manageable units, and tidied-up generally—all in the interests of serving the lecturer's meaning. As with the previous translations of texts by Rudolf Steiner on eurythmy—*Eurythmy as Visible Singing*, *Eurythmy as Visible Speech*, including the early accounts collected in *Eurythmy: Its birth and development*—what has been learned from consultation with colleagues has been assimilated. The aim has been to steer a middle way in adapting an oral style to a written one, yet to preserve the direct freshness of the spoken word.

For this translation, intended in the first place for practising eurythmy therapists, doctors and eurythmists, a few difficult words from the original German text are included within curved brackets ( ). The occasional additions by the translators and by the German and English editors are enclosed in square brackets [ ] in the text, or relegated to footnotes. At the final count, all vagaries and all errors of carelessness and ignorance are to be laid at my door.

Back in 1808, the poet and seminal thinker S.T. Coleridge complained that the medicine of his day was 'too much confined to passive works'. He thought 'a Gymnastic Medicine is wanting' to activate 'the motive faculties'. Steiner's basic impulse to medicine, which includes the inauguration of eurythmy therapy, appeals to the primal, limitless source of healing within every human being.

Alan Stott
Stourbridge, Michaelmas 2008

Pronunciation of some German Sounds

The sounds are given throughout the English text as they are written in original German. The approximate pronunciations are as follows:

A, *ah* as in 'father'
E, *a* as in 'say'
I, *ee* as in 'feet'
O, *oh* as 'load'
U, *oo* as in 'lute'
EI, *i* as in 'light'
AU, *ow* as in 'how'
EU, similar to *oi* as in 'joy', or to Fr. *'jeu'*
V similar to *'f'*

Lecture 1

Dornach, 12 April 1921

During these afternoons, I wish to present the first seeds of a eurythmy therapy. Today I will give a kind of introduction; what we gain from it will be developed into definite forms over the next days. First of all, I would draw attention to some basic matters. What has been practised hitherto is eurythmy as an art;[1] as such it should be accepted along with educational eurythmy suited for children, since what has been developed until now as eurythmy is in every way drawn out of the healthily constituted human being. We will see that certain points can be established. By these means it will be possible to distil from the eurythmical discipline a healthy and therapeutic discipline. It is possible to transform certain artistic forms in one direction or another to become what can be called a eurythmy therapy.

It will be essential, of course, to emphasize that artistic eurythmy—which essentially expresses that element inherent in the formation and tendencies to movement of the human body—is that which has to be deemed correct for the development of the human organism as soul, spirit and body, just as it is appropriate for visual presentation. Yet it is also possible to work towards a eurythmy therapy that will be of extensive use in treating various chronic and acute conditions. It will prove to be especially important and pertinent in those specific cases of impending illnesses and tendencies to illness, which we attempt to treat prophylactically through eurythmy. Here is the point at which the educational element in eurythmy flows gradually over into a healthy and therapeutic activity.

However, for those who wish to practise artistic eurythmy, I want specifically to emphasize that when they do artistic eurythmy they will have thoroughly to forget what they have gained from these present sessions. Precisely in this area we have to maintain a strict separation between those goals which we pursue in health and therapy and that artistic quality which we have to strive to attain in eurythmy. Anyone who persists in mixing the two will first of all ruin his/her artistic ability in eurythmy, and secondly find him/herself unable to achieve anything of importance in respect to its healthy and therapeutic element. Apart from this it will be necessary to acquire some physiological knowledge—which will transform itself into a feeling for the processes forming the human organism—in order to apply the healthy and therapeutic side of eurythmy practically, as we will see in the following lectures.

After these prefatory remarks, I would like to speak more specifically about what may be considered the basis for human eurythmy itself, since it appears to me to be pertinent to the goals we wish to attain. If you wish to understand what eurythmy is in its various aspects, you have first of all to understand the human larynx.[2] We will come to know the other human vocal organs precisely through the series of our exercises relating to the larynx. But the first thing we must obtain will be a certain knowledge of the human larynx and its importance generally for the human organization. There is a much too strong tendency to regard each human organ as a thing unto itself. But that isn't the case; that is not how a human organ lives. Every human organ is a member of the whole organization and, at the same time, a metamorphosed variation of certain other organs. Basically, every self-contained human organ is a metamorphosis of other self-contained human organs. Nevertheless, the case is that certain human organs and groups of organs prove to carry this metamorphic character more exactly within them, more precisely, I would like to say, and others less precisely. The larynx is one organ where you can penetrate through into the essence of the human organism solely through properly understanding metamorphosis.[3]

Recall from your anatomical and physiological knowledge how uniquely the human larynx is formed. What I wish to convey can only be grasped through a Goethean contemplation of the human larynx. You will see that it is possible, if you make the effort to attain this Goethean contemplation of the organs involved, to which we will now direct our attention. Taking the larynx initially as an upwards-directed extension of the windpipe, and studying its forms, you will discover that it may be characterized as a reversed, a from-front-to-back reversed, piece of the human organism—from another place, another piece of the human organization turned around. Picture to yourself the back of the human head, including the auricular parts, and regard what you are picturing to yourself as the back of the human head, including the auricular parts—in so far as these are localized in this part of the human being—excluding the frontal lobe* for the moment, and extending downwards so that it becomes the human rib-cage with its vertebrae, including the beginnings of the ribs which have the much softer breast-bone to the front that lower down falls away altogether. Picture to yourself this less clearly defined system

---

* *Vorderhirn*: literally, the frontal lobe of the brain (tr. note).

of organs that I have presented to you—the posterior part of
the head including the auditory parts, broadening out into
the rib-cage below.

Think now of this part somewhat transformed; imagine the
diameter of the ribs greatly reduced. Imagine that which is
very wide in the ribs, in the rib-cage, here transformed into a
pipe, the bony material being changed into cartilage. Imagine
that part which I isolated as the head to be filled out in such a
way that the less well filled-out parts of the head, those parts
with empty spaces were filled up, and then that which is now
filled in with thicker tissue were left out; think of that which
in the head is actually filled with a liquid-solid mass as
replaced. Imagining the transformation of these parts of the
human organism, you have the metamorphosis of the
larynx—the posterior head with the attached rib-cage,
reversed. The upwards extension into the larynx is truly a
sort of posterior head, transformed. It is actually so; the
etheric formative forces of the larynx bring about an inver-
sion when compared with the formative forces of the above-
mentioned part of the posterior head with the attached rib-
cage. Considering the matter etherically, we carry with the
larynx, in our chest—in a manner of speaking—a second
human being. He—certainly in a rudimentary, stunted
manner, yet in his dispositions, in his stunted beginnings—is
nevertheless at a certain stage of development.

If what I have just described to you were to be returned to
its former position so as to appear as the posterior head, then
in accordance with the formative forces it would of necessity
add on those parts of the forebrain. The tendency to build on
something similar is also present in the larynx. The larynx has
for this reason the thyroid gland in its vicinity.[4] What appears
in more recent physiology as the peculiar conditions of the

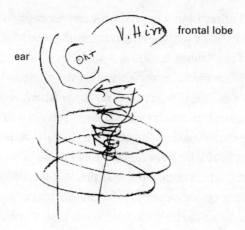

thyroid can be understood in metamorphosis, if you can see a kind of decadent forebrain in the thyroid. This performs functions taken over from the forebrain when someone speaks. The thyroid must cooperate with the frontal lobe. If the thyroid is in any way diseased, you can easily imagine what sort of conditions arise. Simply because he possesses a thyroid, the human being is organized to use it as an organ of thought related more to his chest-nature.

What I have designated as etheric formative forces, which work to bring into being this second human being—who takes up a counter-position in us—these etheric formative forces are actually very differentiated. When we breathe and this breathing expresses itself in speaking or singing, when this modified breathing (for from a certain point of view one must call it that) lives as speech or song, then that whole system of human organs—which I have already indicated as the posterior head continuing down into the chest—is in such inner movement that this movement experiences its reflexes in the organization of the larynx.[5] So, we are to picture to ourselves that this whole system together with the ear is nothing other than a larynx, only metamorphosed—there is a forebrain—this whole system calling forth certain effects which are reflected. Thus our larynx performs eurythmy towards the back, in the form of forces, what we think, feel and so on. This eurythmy really goes on within us. Our larynx eurythmizes. The task is to return that which arises sensory-supersensory through the reflex action of the larynx, to make it visible. Our arms express that which has already been relayed forth and back again. We are dealing here with something taken directly from the human organism.

We have to make it clear to ourselves that we are drawing attention to that organ which has been set into the rhythmic system, like an additional head with a downward extension. Our ordinary head, the more or less thoughtful head, tends to quiet down what pulses up rhythmically into it through the arachnoidal cavity, which is an extension of the breathing.[6] It is by means of the transformation into rest of the movement coming from below into the rhythmic system; thinking is conditioned by virtue of the fact that a state of balance is reached and stasis is developed out of elements in movement, reciprocally conditioning each other in motion—through a static situation arising in the head out of the dynamic situation.

The reverse is also true: what we develop in the rest, in the stasis of the head, influences the dynamic of the rhythmic man, initially in a retarding manner. The fact is that an unnatural exertion of the soul and spirit in connection with the head tends to slow down the circulation. A further consequence is that chaotic or sloppy thinking transforms the rhythmic into the a-rhythmic; it changes the natural rhythm which should play in the human rhythmic system into a-rhythm, even into an anti-rhythm when it comes to full expression. If you wish to understand the human being, you have to observe the connection between the circulatory and respiratory system and careless, chaotic thought, as well as logical thought. Logical thinking as such carries within it the tendency to slow down the rhythm, to make it heavier. Logical thought has the peculiarity of falling out of rhythm. Consequently, the soul-life that wishes to fall into rhythm will try to supersede logic by attempting to frame sentences and verses that follow in their course not the syntax, but the rhythm. By striving to return to rhythm in poetry, by resisting the enemy of poetry—that is prose, with the exception of rhythmical prose, of course—you are trying to become more human. I am *not* claiming that through logic one's development will tend more towards animalism; if you wish, you can always imagine that you evolve towards the angelic level! But in striving to turn from the logical to the human you are trying to bring into the succession of the syllables and their movement, into the movement of the sounds and into the sentence structure, not what is demanded by the syntax but that which the rhythm requires. We pay heed to the rhythmic man when wanting to return to the realm of poetry; we listen to the headman when wishing to enter into prose.

This will serve to indicate the connection actually existing between that manifest part of man, which I have described, and that part which, as a metamorphosis of it, is somewhat concealed. He is there within us, however, this eurythmist who as the etheric body of the larynx performs a distinct eurythmy intimately connected with the normal development of our respiratory system, with our whole circulatory system and, naturally, through the intermediary of the circulatory system even with the metabolic system—as you can surmise from all that I have presented.

Now, all possible sorts of occasions arise for this very complicated arrangement, this dovetailing of a forward-orientated and a backward-orientated system, to become disjointed. It would be accurate to say that this is properly knit together only in very few people in today's culture. It will be necessary to develop a certain ability to observe this. When the head-system, for example, has been so dealt with in childhood that the transgression against the rhythmic system is too great, everything possible can develop in later years simply through an irregularity in what I have described. This is precisely because in the case of the human organism, as in an avalanche, small provocations may build up great effects.

In observing children from this aspect you will find that it is extremely significant to what degree their unconscious living in rhythm predominates in their soul-life over the quieting element of the head-organization. For example, if this is the case, if the rhythmic system predominates, you must ask yourself whether something should not be introduced into the education of the child. If in time the condition appears to be habitual, then something must be done. When, as a result of the anomaly to which I have drawn attention, the child becomes increasingly excited, ever more and more fluttery and nothing can be done with him, you must attempt to bring an iambic element into his whole organization. This can be done by having the child move in such a manner that, in full consciousness—for that he must receive your guidance—he moves first the left arm and the left hand forwards, then the right arm, so that this becomes more conscious. The child is aware: that is the first and was the first. Throughout the entire exercise the consciousness must prevail: that was the first and remains the first; it began with the left. One can reinforce the whole affair by having the child walk, stepping out with the left leg and bringing the right leg up to it, so that the leg-and-foot exercise is added to the hand-and-arm exercise, but only to reinforce. (This can be practised tomorrow[7] in connection with something else.) The arm-exercise is really the essential thing. If one has the child practise in this iambic manner, as one may call it, one will see that the exercises will calm the fluttery child, the excited child, and so on, provided they are continued over a sufficiently long period of time.

Out of your knowledge of eurythmy you could describe it like this. You have the child do half an 'A' with the left arm and then complete this half-'A' to a whole 'A' with the right arm, and so on, so that the child remains in motion and the 'A' does not come into being all at once, but as the result of successive movements.

If on the other hand you have a child who is phlegmatic, who doesn't want to take things in (our Waldorf teachers know these children well, they can at times bring one to a mild despair), these children actually hear nothing of what one says to them; everything passes them by. In this case, one would do well to treat this child trochaically, that is to say, in just the opposite manner. Naturally, one cannot begin with everything all at once; this is an element which has yet to be brought into Waldorf education.[8] You form the 'A' so that the child knows: first the right arm, then the left arm, right arm, left arm and then further that first the right leg is placed in front and the left leg brought up to it; thus one has the arm movements forming the 'A' (one after the other) reinforced by the leg-and-foot movement. Pay particular attention that these things are done in such a way that they live in the child's consciousness, so that the child is really aware: on one occasion the left arm was the first, on the other the right arm was the first.

You will find that these things present difficulties for an inner understanding for someone who in every way is a physiologist in the modern sense, believing that man's whole soul-life is mediated through the nervous system. That is, those who do not know that feeling is mediated by the rhythmic system, the will by the metabolic system, and that only thought formation is mediated by the nervous system. If you do not know these things you will have great difficulty in grasping the significance of what happens in any part of the body, both in respect to the soul and spirit part and to the bodily part of the human being.

The person who has developed an ability to observe knows that when a person makes clumsy hand and finger movements, and so on, he will exhibit a particular manner of thinking as well that can be compared with what happens in the fingers. It is really extremely interesting to study the connection between the manner in which a person controls the mechanics of the arm and the finger-physiognomy with the way he thinks. For the qualities of soul and spirit which a person portrays proceed from the whole human being, not solely from the brain and nervous tissue. We have to learn to understand that we think not only with the brain but also with the little finger and the big toe.[9] There is a certain significance in achieving lightness—particularly in the limbs—as this will bring lightness into the soul-life as well. These ideas will only become applicable (as we shall see in the following lectures) when we are given the possibility of providing a truly complete school hygiene to accompany the other teaching. It can happen, for example, that a child is peculiarly unable to comprehend geometrical figures. He cannot understand a geometrical figure by looking at it.[10] However difficult it may be, you will do this child a great service by making him take a small pencil between the big toe and the next toe, and write really proper letters. That is something which carries a specific significance and which points in a fully justified manner to an interrelationship in man.

Especially in the case of children, one may notice that the three members of the human organization do not, as it were, click properly into one another. A really large part of the anomalies of life are due to this improper articulation. To begin with, children experience headaches;[11] at the same time one notices that the digestion is disturbed, and so on. The most varied conditions may appear. We will give further indications in this regard in conjunction with other exercises to be shown in the next days. However, when confronted with a situation such as I have described you can achieve a great deal with the child or children through having them do the following exercise: a eurythmical 'I' (as you already know), a eurythmical 'A' and a eurythmical 'O', but so that the children do the 'I' with the whole upper body. For our physician friends I want to emphasize particularly that what is essential in eurythmy—and that through which one achieves what is essential in artistic eurythmy as well—is not the mere form of the limb in position seen from without, but that which comes into being when the stretching or the bending within the positioned limb is *felt*. What is felt in the limb is what is important. Assume that you do an 'I' with both arms; this 'I' will not appear as it should when seen from without if you observe only its line, its content as a form. You must feel concurrently; you can tell by looking at the person that he feels the stretching power in the 'I' as he does it. Similarly,

when a person does, for example, an 'E' the important thing
is not that he does this (crosses the arms), but that he feels:
here one limb comes to rest on the other. In this feeling of
one limb on the other lies the 'E' in reality; what you see is the
expression for this sensing of one limb through the other.
Then what you *do* here is no different from what you do when
you *look*. You are continually carrying out an 'E' by crossing
the axis of the right eye with the axis of the left in order to find
a point and so arrive [at a crossing].[12] That is actually 'the
primal E'; what has been demonstrated here is basically an
imitation of it. Yet everything in man is a metamorphosis,
and this is a perfectly justifiable imitation, as in speaking 'E'
the larynx carries out in the etheric exactly the same form to
the rear.

$$I A O$$

When you practise this exercise with a child it is necessary
that the 'I' be done with the upper body, that is to say, the
child stretches out his upper body. He feels the whole body
stretched. He does the 'A' with his legs and the 'O' by moving
his arms like this. Have the child do the following as quickly
as possible in sequence: stretch the upper body vertically,
separate the legs, and do the 'O'-movement with the arms;
release and repeat, release and repeat, and so on. One can
practise such a thing with the children in chorus, of course.
However, in principle such exercises should not be practised
with the children as a class. Artistic eurythmy and the
eurythmy for educational and instructive reasons should be
done by a class as a whole, for here children of the same age

belong together. In order to make the transition from the usual class-eurythmy to these matters related to health-stimulating and therapeutic eurythmy, in order to practise with them one must take those children who need such an exercise out of various classes, due to the peculiarities which I have described—the disharmony of the three members of the human organism. One can take them out of the most varied classes and then practise this exercise with those particularly suited for it. That really must be done if one truly wishes to pursue a eurythmy for health, a therapeutic eurythmy, in the school. Thus we are already on the path which, as we follow it further, will lead us to study certain movements that are actually only metamorphoses of the usual eurythmical movements and to trace their effect on the human organization. The fact is that we have interior organs with certain forms. These forms may be subject to anomalies. The form of each organ stands in a certain relationship to a possible form of movement of the outer man. So the following may be said. Let us assume that some organ, let's say the gall bladder, tends towards deformation, a tendency to assume an abnormal form. A form of movement exists which will counteract this tendency. Such is the case with every organ. It is in this direction that we intend to develop what will follow. What I have given today was meant as an introduction to guide you to the path leading into this subject.

Lecture 2

Dornach, 13 April 1921

Today I intend to discuss matters related to the vowel element in eurythmy.[13] We need only to recall—as it is known to us through spiritual science—that vowels express more that which lives inwardly in the human being as feelings, emotions, and so on. Consonants describe more that which is outwardly objective. When we remain within the realm of speech, these two statements are valid: vowels, more expression, revelation of the inwardness of feeling; we reveal ourselves to an extent in the vowel, that is to say, we reveal what we feel towards an object. Through the movements that the tongue, the lips and the palate perform, the consonants conform themselves more sculpturally to the outward forms of objects—as they are spiritually experienced, of course—and attempt to reconstruct them. Basically all the consonants are more reproductions of the outward form of things. However, we can actually only speak of vowels and consonants in this manner when we have in mind an earlier stage of human evolution. At that earlier time of the evolution of speech, the movement of the whole body and of the limbs as well was self-evident—since the individual sounds were always to a degree connected with movements of the body. This connection has been loosened in the course of human development. Speech was taken more towards the interior; the possibilities of movement, of expression through movement, ceased. Today in normal life we speak largely without accompanying our speech with the corresponding movements. In eurythmy, we bring back the movements attending the vowels and consonants, so bringing the body into movement again. Now, we have to realize that when we utter vowels we omit the movement that previously joined in the outer movement and we make the vowel inward. We take something away from it on its path inwards. We take the movement away. We restore to the vowel in outer movement what we have taken away from it on its inward-going path. In the case of the vowel, matters are such that the outward movement is of exceptional importance in the search for the transition into the effective working of the vowel, eurythmically expressed, on to the whole human being. That is what we take into account here.

In speaking of vowels today, we will speak purely of the meaning of that which is eurythmically vocalized in movement. Here it is very important that we develop a feeling for what flows into the movement. We develop a perceptive consciousness that tells us whether what is happening in the respective human limb is a stretching, a rounding, or some such. One must decidedly acquire a specific consciousness for this. In what pertains to vowels, it is extremely important to feel the movement made or the position taken up. That is what is important. Starting from here, we will transpose each of the vowels from the eurythmical into the therapeutic aspect.

Practically demonstrated (Frau Baumann): a distinct 'I' (*ee*) made by stretching both arms. This stretching should be carried out in such a way that you then return [to the rest position] and perform the same movement somewhat lower, return again, doing it with both arms horizontal. Now we go back and, if you had the right arm forward at first, now, as you go lower, you must take the right to the back, and now to the front, now a bit back again, and then somewhat deeper. Now I don't want to strain you further with that, but if you wanted to carry it out, you could make it more complicated by taking more positions. You would then start with the 'I', return, do it a little further on, go back, a little further on, and so forth, so that one has as many 'I'-positions as possible, carried out from above to below, always returning [to the rest position]. When these movements are performed, they are an expression for the human being as a person. The entire individual person is thereby expressed.

Now we could notice, for example, that some child—for that matter an adult—cannot express himself properly as a person. He is somehow inhibited in expressing himself as a complete individuality. He might be a dreamer in a certain sense, or something similar. Or, if we think of a physical abnormality—in the case of a child, for example, that hasn't learnt to walk properly, he walks clumsily. Or if in the case of an adult we notice that it would be desirable for reasons of health or therapy that a person learns to walk better, this particular exercise would be very good for this. When adults step out too little in their stride, when they don't reach out properly with their steps, it always means that the circulation suffers from it. The circulation of the blood suffers under an insufficiently outreaching gait. So when people walk in this way [lightly tripping], that has the consequence that the circulation becomes in some fashion slower than it should be in that person. Attempt to have this person learn to step out again, and by having him do this exercise, you will be certain to attain your goal. Then the person will have greater and more penetrating results in learning to walk properly. So we can say that in essence this modified 'I'-exercise furthers those people who—I will express it somewhat radically—

cannot walk properly. It can be summed up approximately like this—for people who cannot walk properly.

You can extend the exercise further, and, with the addition of a sort of resumée of what Frau Baumann has done, it will be that much more effective. Now try to do the whole 'I'-exercise without bringing the arms back [to the rest position], so that you reach the last position only by turning—turning in a plane, quick, quicker and even quicker. The 'I'-exercise as it was first demonstrated and described can be intensified in this way and will benefit those people who cannot walk properly. It will then be extraordinarily easy to bring them to walk properly. One can admonish them to walk properly, and their efforts to walk in a different manner will bring suitable results as well.

Now Frau Baumann will demonstrate an 'U'-exercise for us. The arms quite high up, and back to the starting position, now a little lower, back again, a little lower, now horizontal, back again, now below, back again, and again below; that is the principle of it. And now do it straightaway so that you start above maintaining the 'U' as you move downwards; and now do it increasingly quickly so that at last you reach quite a speed.

Please keep this in mind as the manner in which to execute the 'U'-exercise. If I were to summarize again in the same fashion as earlier, I would call this the movement for children or adults who cannot stand. In the case of 'I' we had those who cannot walk, with 'U', we have those who cannot stand.

Now, not being able to stand is to have weak feet and to become very easily tired when standing. It would also mean, for example, that one could not stand long enough on tiptoe properly, or that one could not stand on one's heels long enough without immediately becoming clumsy. Standing on tiptoe or on the heels are not eurythmical exercises, but they should be practised by people who have weak legs, who tire easily while standing or who can't stand properly at all. To be unable to stand properly is to be easily tired in walking as well. That is a technical difference; to walk awkwardly and to tire in walking are two different things. When a person is tired by walking, one has to do the 'U'-exercise. When a person walks clumsily or when as a result of his whole constitution it would be desirable for him to learn to step out with his feet, that can be technically expressed as being unable to walk. However, to be tired by walking would be technically expressed as not being able to stand. For such people the 'U'-exercise is especially appropriate. This is interrelated with matters with which we can deal once we have gone a little further.

Now please do the 'O'-movement: quite high up and then back [to the rest position] and now somewhat lower, back again, lower still, and so on. Now do it so that you do the 'O'-movement above; feel distinctly the rounding of the arms within the movement as you glide down. When you glide down with the 'O'-movement it must remain an 'O'. Then ever quicker and quicker.

You would see this exercise complete in its most brilliant application, my friends, if you had here in front of you a really corpulent person. If a child or adult becomes unnaturally fat, then this is the exercise to be applied. By making the 'O' so often and by extending it to this barrel-shaped body at the end—for it really is a barrel one describes outside oneself—we in fact carry out that which forms the opposite pole to those dynamic tendencies at work in making a person obese. It can be applied very well for health and therapy, and you will be convinced that a tendency to become thinner actually appears when you have such people carry out this movement, especially when they practise other things as well which we have yet to discuss. But at the same time in this exercise it is of special significance that you have the person practise only as long as he/she can without sweating heavily and becoming too warm. If you wish to attain the desired effect, you must try to conduct the exercise so that the person can always rest in between.

Now Frau Baumann will perhaps be so kind as to do an 'E'-movement, quite high above. It is a proper 'E'-movement only when this hand lies on the other so that they touch. Now return [to the rest position], then somewhat lower, the right hand over the left arm, and then, so that it is really effective, we will do it so that it lies increasingly further back and now again from above to below; then the 'E' must be done so that it penetrates thoroughly. And now, in bringing it down, you move further back, so far that you split the shoulder seam at the back. Now this is the exercise that will be especially advantageous for weaklings, that is to say, for thin folk rather than fat folk, for those people in whom the weakness comes distinctly from within but is organically conditioned. It has to be organically caused.

Another exercise which can be considered parallel to this should be applied with some caution as it affects the soul more closely. It is the following. Do an 'E' to the rear as well as you can and as far in as you can. That really hurts. It is a movement that is in itself a little painful, and that is indeed the purpose. It should be practised with those children or adults in whom there are psychological grounds for becoming thin, such as becoming worn down, and so on. Since you must in principle be careful in approaching from the outside with therapy by such spiritual means, this too must of course be applied with caution. That means that one attempts to engage moral impulses when working with a child who is faint-hearted or who shows signs of depression, when you let him do these exercises. If one concerns oneself with the child otherwise by comforting him and caring for his soul, then you can have him do these exercises as well.

You can see that in the case of all these things it is to a degree a matter of extending what comes to expression in artistic eurythmy. This is especially true in respect to the vowels.

Now it is very important that we make the following clear to ourselves. You know that the vowel-element can be developed in this fashion, and that in essence it expresses inner experience. One must only grasp through feeling and contemplation what takes place. Bear in mind that the person concerned, the person who carries out these things in order to enter therapy, feels them. In 'E' he feels that one arm covers the other. In the case of 'O', though, something more comes into consideration. In 'O', feel not only the closing of the circle, but the bending as well. You feel that you are forming a circle. Feel the circle that runs through it. And in order to make the 'O' particularly effective, make the person doing it aware, too, that he should feel as though he himself or someone else were to draw a line along his breastbone. By means of feeling, the whole is closed to the rear in spirit—as if one were to experience something like having a line drawn on the breastbone by oneself or someone else.

Now we want to do an 'A': return [to the rest position], we do an 'A' somewhat lower, return again, do an 'A' horizontally, return, do an 'A' somewhat lowered, return, an 'A' very deep, return, then to the rear; this you need to do only once, but return first [to the rest position]. And now do the 'A' above and without changing the angle lead it down, and to the back, again without feeling that you change the angle.

This exercise can be really effective only if you have it done frequently. And when you have it repeated frequently, it is the exercise to be used with people who are greedy, in whom the animal nature comes particularly strongly to the fore. So if you have in school children who are in every way proper little animals and in whom the condition has an organic cause, when you have them do this exercise you will see that it has for them a very particular significance.

In the case of these exercises you can observe once again that if they are to be introduced into the school it will be necessary to organize the children into groups especially for them. You will soon become convinced that the children do these exercises much less gladly than the other eurythmical exercises. While they are eager to do the others, you will most likely have to persuade them to do these, as they will react at first as children often react to taking medicine—with resistance. They won't be particularly happy about it, but that is of no especial harm in the exercises having to do with 'O', 'U', 'E' and 'A'. In the case of 'I' it is somewhat harmful when the child doesn't enjoy it. You must try to reach the stage where the children delight in the 'I'-exercise as we have done it. In the case of the others 'U', 'O' 'E' and 'A', it is not especially damaging if they carry out the exercise on authority, and knowing that it is their duty to do it. With 'I' it is important that the children enjoy doing it as it affects the whole individual, as I have already said.

You will profit further by coming to terms with the following. The 'I' reveals man as a person; the 'U' reveals man as man; the 'O' reveals man as soul; the 'E' fixes the ego in the etheric body, it strongly penetrates the etheric body with the ego. And the 'A' counteracts the animal-nature in man.

Now we will follow the various effects further. If you have a person with irregular breathing, who is in some fashion burdened down by his breathing and suchlike, you will be able to bring this person to normal breathing by applying the vowels. You will be able to achieve in particular the distinct articulation of the consonants by means of these exercises, as that is greatly facilitated through the practice of the vowels. When you notice that certain children cannot manage to form certain consonants with the lips or the tongue—for the palate sounds it is less applicable, although for the labial and lingual sounds exceptionally good—it will be of great help to the children with difficulties in this respect when one tries to have them do such vowel exercises as early as possible.[14]

You will also notice that when people tend to chronic headaches, to migraine-like conditions,[15] these can be appreciably alleviated through the practice of the vowels. So in the cases of chronic headaches and chronic migraine symptoms, as well as when people are foggy-headed, these things will be particularly applicable. Similarly, if you employ the exercises that we have done today for certain children who cannot pay attention, who are sleepy, you will awaken them in a certain sense to a state of awareness. That is a healthy and instructive angle of a certain significance. It will be observed that sleepy-headed adults can also be awakened in this way. And then one will notice that when a person's digestion is too weak or too slow that by means of these exercises this slow digestion and all that is known to be connected with it can be changed for the better.

In certain forms of health-promoting-eurythmy it would be good to have the movements—which are carried out with

the arms only in artistic eurythmy—carried out with the legs
as well where possible, only somewhat less forcefully, as I am
about to describe. Now, you will ask how one can do an 'I',
for example, with the legs? It's very easy. One must only
stretch out the leg and feel the stretching in it. The 'U' would
be simply to stand with full awareness on both legs, so that
one has a distinct feeling of stretching in both. 'O' with the
legs, though, must be learned. One should really accustom
the people with whom one finds it necessary to do the 'O'-
exercise in the manner that I have described to do the 'O'
with the legs as well. That consists in pointing the toes
somewhat, but only very slightly, to the outside and then
trying to stand in this manner, holding one's position. One
must thereby stand on tiptoe, however, and bend outward,
remain so standing a moment and then return to the normal
position; then build it up again, and so on.

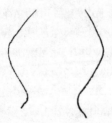

It is necessary to take into account the relationship existing
between the possibilities of organically determined inner
movement for the middle man and the lower man. This is
such that movement done for the lower man should be carried out at only one-third the strength. So when you have
someone carry out the 'O'-movement as we have seen it, feel
that what is done later for the legs and feet requires only one-
third of the time and thus only a third of the energy

expended. It will be especially effective, however, when you place this in the middle, so that you have a third, a third and a third, let us say, 'A' and then 'A' again, with 'B' as foot movement in the middle (see the table); it will be particularly effective to have them together—a third, a third and a third; that will be particularly effective.

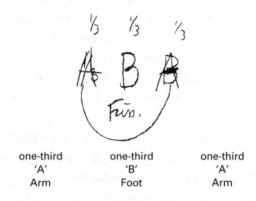

one-third	one-third	one-third
'A'	'B'	'A'
Arm	Foot	Arm

It will also be especially effective to do the same in connection with the 'E'-exercise for the feet, by really crossing the feet. But one must stand on tiptoe and place one leg over the other so that they touch. Again, one-third, and if possible placed in the middle. That is something which it would be particularly good to have done by children and by adults as well who are weaklings. They will naturally be hardly capable of doing it, but that is exactly why they must learn to do it. In precisely these matters you see that what is most important for various people to learn is what they are most incapable of doing. They must learn it because it is necessary to the recovery of their health.

'A' [with the legs] is also necessary; I demonstrated it to you yesterday. It consists in assuming this spread position while standing, in so far as it is possible on tiptoe. That

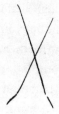

should also be introduced into the 'A'-movement and it will be particularly effective there.

Now, one can also intensify all the exercises that we have just described by carrying them out in walking. And you will achieve a great deal for a weak child, for example, when you teach him to do the 'E'-motion as we have just done it, in walking; he should walk in such a manner that he always touches each leg alternately. In taking a step forward he crosses over first with one leg, then with the other, so that he always crosses one leg over the other, so that he places one leg behind and touches it with the other in front. Naturally he won't move ahead very well, but it is good to have this movement carried out while walking. You will say that complicated movements appear as a result; but it is good when complicated movements appear.

Now I want to bring it to your attention that what we have said about the vowel element should initially be sharply distinguished from what we will practise tomorrow in respect to the consonants. The consonantal element is such that it generally expresses the external, as we have already said. In speech as well, the consonant is so formed that a reconstruction, an imitation of the outer form comes into being through the formative motions of lips and tongue. Now, as we shall see tomorrow, the consonants have very special sorts of movements. It lies within these forms of movement to

make the consonant inward again in a certain manner by
giving it eurythmical form. It is internalized. That which it
loses in the outward-going path of speech is restored to it.
And, whether one is contemplating them in eurythmy as art
or performing them for personal reasons, in the case of
consonants it is particularly important to have, not a feeling
in the way one does with a vowel, a feeling of stretching, of
bending, or of widening and so on, but to imagine oneself
simultaneously in the form that one carries out while doing
the consonants, as though one were to observe oneself.

Here you can see most clearly that we must admonish
the artistic eurythmists *not* to mix up the two things; the
artistic eurythmists would not do well to observe themselves constantly as they would rob themselves of their
ability to work unselfconsciously. On the contrary, when
you have a child or a grown-up carry out something having
to do with consonants, it is important that they, as it were,
photograph themselves inwardly in their thought; then in
this inward photographing of oneself lies that which is
effective. The person must really see himself inwardly in
the position that he is carrying out; it has to be carried out
in such a manner that the person makes an inner picture of
what he does.

If you would be so good (Frl. Wolfram) as to show us an
'M' as a consonant, first with the right hand, now with the
left, but taking it backwards, now taking the right hand back,
and 'M' with the left hand and now with both hands, that can
be multiplied in various ways, of course. Now an 'M', we will
start with this example to begin with: what is it as speech? In
speech 'M' is an extraordinarily important sound. You will
experience its importance in speech, and in speech physiology as well, by contrasting it with the 'S'. Perhaps Frau

Baumann will do a graceful 'S' for us now, right, left, and now with both hands.

Now to begin with it appears that you have the feeling, or feel when the 'S' is done,[16] that you move something within you. It is the etheric body [at this point the lecturer made the corresponding movement]; you move so that you have a snakelike line. This serpentine may approach a straight line in the case of a particularly sharply pronounced 'S' and can even be represented as a straight line.

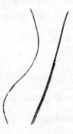

By contrast, when you look at the 'M' that was just performed, you have to feel—even when the organic form in which it is carried out is similar—it is not exactly the same element, it is linearly not the same. And so the 'M' is that which, laid against the 'S'-direction, counters the 'S'-direction. This basically is the great contrast between the 'S' and the 'M'. 'S' and 'M' are the two polar sounds. 'S' is the truly ahrimanic sound, if I may speak anthroposophically, and the 'M' is that which mitigates the ahrimanic properties, makes it mild; if I may express it so, it takes its ahrimanic strength from it. So, when we have a combination of sounds directly including 'S' and 'M', for example *Samen*, 'seeds', or *Summe*, 'sum', we have in this combination of sounds first the strong ahrimanic being in the 'S', whose sting is then taken from it by the 'M'.

Will you show us an 'H' (Frl. Wolfram)? When you really look at the 'H', when you feel yourself really within this 'H', then, you will say to yourself, there is something in this 'H' which reveals itself as unequivocally luciferic. It is the luciferic in the 'H', then, which comes to expression here. Try to observe yourself—here the feeling is less important than the observation of it. Try to observe it yourself, when Frau Baumann does it for us now, how it is when one does the 'H' and allows it to go over immediately into an 'M'. Do the 'H' first and by and by let it carry over into an 'M'. Now take a look at it. In this movement you have the whole perception of the mitigation of the luciferic, of its sting being taken from it, brought to expression. The movement is truly as if one would stop Lucifer. And one can also hear it if you simply think about it—the civilized person today can actually no longer reflect properly on these things. If someone wants to agree to something luciferic, but immediately diminishes the actual luciferic element, the eagerness of his assent, then he says, 'Hm, hm'. There you have the 'H' and the 'M' placed really very close to one another; you have the whole charm of the diminished luciferic directly within it.

From this, you can see that as soon as you turn to the consonantal element you must immediately turn to the observation of the form as well. That is the essential thing; tomorrow we will speak about it further.

Lecture 3

Dornach, 14 April 1921

In order to proceed in an appropriate manner, we will prepare the ground today for certain matters to be deepened physiologically and psychologically tomorrow, by considering the forms which consonants take in eurythmical movement. In what has been developed as the form involved in consonantal movement, consideration has been truly given to everything that has to be taken into account when you attempt to penetrate into the outer world through speech. The person who sets himself the task of observing speech will see that man's confrontation with the outer world consists on the one hand of vigorously living into the world, of making himself selfless and living into the world. In the vowels he comes to himself; in the vowels he goes within and unfolds his activity there. In the consonants he becomes in a way one with the outer world, although to varying degrees. These varying degrees of unification with the world are manifest in certain practices within language as well. In the development of the consonantal element in eurythmy, particularly in reference to the sensory-supersensory observation (of which I so often speak[17] in introducing eurythmy performances), it is necessary to consider whether the human being objectifies himself. We have to discover whether in a spoken sound a man objectifies himself completely in order to lay hold of the spiritual element in the things outside him or if, despite this objectification of himself, he remains more within—not going completely out of himself but instead reproducing the external within himself. That is a major distinction, by reason of which I must ask Frau Baumann to be so good and show us first of all the movement for 'H'. Now, please disregard this 'H'-movement altogether, and Frau Baumann will demonstrate the 'F'-movement. Now, keep an eye on what you can observe here in these two different movements. You can observe what is present by virtue of the human instinct in the attempt to enunciate the sound in question. Consider the pronunciation of 'H'—you actually say *Ha*, you follow up with a vowel. It is impossible to sound a consonant without it being tinged by a vowel; you follow it up with an 'A'. The pure consonant is vocalized, combined with a vowel. If you consider the 'F', you will find that our linguistic instinct places an 'E' in front of it: '*eF*.' Here the opposite occurs; an 'E' is set before it.

ha ef

Through the foregoing you will perceive that when a man utters an 'H'-sound, he makes a greater effort to uncover through speech the spiritual element in the external object; when he utters an 'F'-sound his effort is directed more towards re-experiencing the spiritual within himself. Consequently, the manner in which the consonant arises is entirely different, according to whether the vowel tinges the consonant from the front or from the back—if I may use this manner of expression in respect to the nature of consonantal articulation. This you will find conveyed in the form you have observed.

Perhaps Frl. Wolfram will do the 'H' once again. 'H': here you have an energetic unfolding into the outer world; one doesn't wish to remain in oneself, one wants to go out and live in the external world. 'F': you see the decided effort to avoid entering into the outer world too sharply, to remain in the inner experience.

Now when we takes this into consideration, we can carry on from here to form an idea of various matters which, although they are to become part of eurythmy, were initially unnecessary as far as we have been concerned with eurythmy as an art, but which will become necessary the more this art is extended to other languages. The moment one says not *ef* but *fi* it is a different matter; in that moment one attempts to embrace the external with the sound as well. This is indicative of an important historical fact. In ancient Greece people attempted to grasp the external, even in those things in respect to which our contemporaries have become inward. You see how you can follow into the outermost fringes of man's experience what I have expressed, for example, in my book *The Riddles of Philosophy*,[18] this going out and taking hold in the external world of what man today already experiences entirely inwardly in his 'I', his ego. The reason why spiritual science is not accepted because of such facts is solely because the people of our civilization are generally too lazy. They have to take too many things into account in order to come to the truth, and they want to make it easier for themselves. But that just won't do! They want to make everything easier for themselves, and that won't do.

That, for the present, in respect to one element which flowed into the formation of the consonants. If we want to understand the formation of consonants in the realm of eurythmy, then we should consider a second element to which I believe people pay less attention nowadays in teaching, even in physiology, speech physiology, than the third element which we will come to in a moment. In order to form an impression, I will ask you to compare once again. Here it is important that you form a contemplative picture. Naturally, one cannot penetrate to the very end of what one has in such a picture, to the concept.

Perhaps Frau Baumann will be so good and do the 'H' again, and once the tone has faded away Frau Baumann will do a 'D' for us. Pay attention in this case to the following. When you contemplate the 'H' you will find the movement for it initially deviates greatly from what takes place in speaking it, since—in respect to the characteristic of which I am thinking at the moment—the eurythmical element has to stand as polar opposite to the actual process in speech. You know that the speech process, as I presented it the day before yesterday, is a reflecting back from the larynx. The eurythmical process must express this outwardly. It expresses it in movement. In certain instances one must go over to the exactly opposite pole. This is particularly characteristic of 'H' and 'D'; in the case of other consonants this element has to be toned down. Now, what sort of a sound is 'H'? 'H' is essentially a breath sound. The 'H' is actually brought into being through blowing—where you have to blow in speaking, you have to make a decided, shoving thrust. When you utter 'D' you have this thrusting effect in the pronunciation. [In eurythmy] we must polarize this by transforming it into the characteristic movement that is present in 'D'. Here the thrusting quality of speech is lamed when one conveys the sound through movement.

So you see that precisely this characteristic has to be taken particularly into account, when we have either a breath sound or a plosive sound.[19] Now, sounds are not only either breath sounds or plosives. But by what reason are they one or the other? You see, when one has a decided breath sound, one expresses by means of the blowing the fact that one really wants to go out of oneself. One expresses in the thrusting that this going out of oneself is difficult, that one would like to remain within. For this reason the eurythmical transposition of the sound has to take place in the manner you have seen.

Now, there are also sounds that carefully connect the inward with the outward; sounds that are actually physiologically so constituted that with them one states that one is bringing to a standstill, arresting, that in which one would like to be active in such a manner that the inward would immediately become outward, where one would enter into the movement immediately with the whole human being. This is decidedly evident in only one sound in our language, the 'R'. It is, however, for this reason the most inclusive sound. When you say 'R' you would like to run after the speech organism with every limb, as I would like to express it. Actually, with 'R' one strives to bring this pursuit to rest. The lips want to follow when they pronounce the labial 'R', and bring this 'running-after' to a halt. The tongue wants to follow when it speaks the lingual 'R', and finally the palate wants to follow when the palatal 'R' sounds. These three 'R's are distinctly different from one another, but are nevertheless one; in eurythmy they are expressed thus (Fr. Baumann: 'R'). The bringing-into-swing of what one usually brings to a standstill is expressed. It is precisely the running after the movement of the sound that is expressed in the 'R'. And when you want to express the other element, you can express the labial 'R' by carrying the movement further downwards; the lingual 'R' can be made more in the horizontal, and the palatal 'R' rather more upwards. By this means one can modify the 'R'-sound in the eurythmical movement. But you see that the form is determined by leaving the vibration of the 'R' in the background and expressing the 'running-after'.

The 'L' (Frl. Wolfram: 'L') is a similar sound where we have, not a vibrating, but a sort of wave in the movement. You see that there is something of the same movement in it as in the 'R', but the 'running-after' is gentle and comes to rest. It is a wave rather than a vibration that comes to expression.

That is what is connected inwardly, physiologically, with the shading through the vowel element of the consonantal sound, and with the shading through feeling, which already leads to a greater extent into the physical. We arrive at the outermost division of the sounds[20] by considering the organs. If once again we compare the respective movements we will arrive at the most outward, the most external principles of division through our contemplative picture (Fr. Baumann: 'B'). That is a 'B', and now we will continue directly perhaps with a 'T' [Fr. Baumann: 'T']. Now you can see from the position—which as the third element must be taken into account and which makes itself quite apparent to sensory-supersensory contemplation—that in the case of 'B' we are dealing with a labial sound and in the case of 'T' with a dental sound (Frl. Wolfram, please do a 'K' for us). 'K': here one starts with the position and the essential lies in the movement. Here we have to do with a palatal sound which in its pronunciation, in the tone in which it is spoken, is the quietest, but which has to be transformed in movement into its polar opposite when performed outwardly in eurythmy. The consonants overlap in respect to their characteristics;

one division extends into another. The following may serve as an aid.

Take the labial sounds—I will write out only the most distinctive of them: 'W [= V]', 'B', 'P', 'F', 'M'. You can determine to what extent the vowel colouring is involved by pronouncing the sounds; I don't need to indicate that. Let us take the dental sounds 'D', 'T', 'S', 'Sh', 'L', the English 'Th', and 'N'. And now the palatal sounds: 'G', 'K', 'Ch', and the French 'Ng', more or less. We will have to write the 'R' in everywhere, since it has its nuances everywhere:

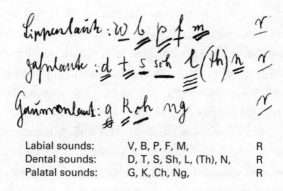

Labial sounds:	V, B, P, F, M,	R
Dental sounds:	D, T, S, Sh, L, (Th), N,	R
Palatal sounds:	G, K, Ch, Ng,	R

Considering the process of division from the other point of view now, I will underline with white where we have to do with a definite breath sound: 'V', 'F', 'S', 'Sh' and 'Ch' as well, more or less. These would be the decided breath sounds. I will underline in red where we have to do with what are clearly plosives: 'B', 'P', 'M', 'D', 'T', 'N', and then perhaps 'G' and 'K'. The vibratory sound is 'R'. We have to do with a distinct undulating sound—which, because of the soft transformation in the movement, must be in a sense of an inward character—fundamentally only in the case of 'L'.

These three organizational principles—the vowel colouring, the blowing, thrusting, vibrating and undulating, and all that which has to do with the external division [into dental, labial and palate sounds]—all this comes to expression in the forms given for eurythmy. It must be clear to you, of course, to what degree these principles of division affect each other. With 'L', for example, we have to do with a distinct dental sound which must have all the characteristics of a dental sound. Then, having to do with a gliding sound, with an undulant sound, it must have the characteristics of a wave. Apart from that, it has a strong connection to the inward. We have to do with a colouring from within outwards, at least in our language. We don't say *le*, but *el*; here we have the transition from earlier forms, in which people reached yearningly into the exterior world. As a result, a word [Lambda, the eleventh letter of the Greek alphabet] was used in order to express such an event, in order to bring this going over into the external to proper expression. Thus in each of the letters we have to do with a picture of that which is taking place inwardly.

Before we consider the consonants individually, let us contemplate the following. Yesterday we were able to show that 'A'—which we also studied in its metamorphosis—has to do with all those forces in man that make him greedy, which organize him according to animal nature: the 'A' in fact lies nearest to the animal nature in man, and in a certain sense one can say that when the 'A' is pronounced it sounds out of the animality of man. And certainly as spiritual investigation confirms 'A' is the sound that was the very earliest to appear in the course of both the phylogentic evolution as well as the ontogenetic evolution of man. In ontogenetic evolution it is somewhat hidden of course; there is a false evolution as well, as you know. The 'A' was the first sound to appear in humankind's evolution, resounding initially, however, entirely out of the animal nature. And when we tend towards 'A' with the consonants, we are still calling on what are animal forces in man. As you could see yesterday, the whole sound is actually formed accordingly. If we use the sound therapeutically in the manner in which it presented itself to our souls yesterday we can combat that which makes children, and grown-ups too, into smaller and larger animals. With such exercises we can have very respectable results in the de-animalization of man.[21]

And now let us go on to the sound 'U', for example. We said yesterday that this is the sound we use therapeutically when a person cannot stand. You saw that yesterday. It is the sound which in a certain respect expresses its physiological-pathological connection already in the manner in which it is formed in speech. The 'U' is spoken with the mouth and the openings between the teeth constricted to the greatest degree and with the lips somewhat extended, in such a way, however, that the mouth opening is narrowed and the lips can vibrate. You can see that in speaking one seeks an essentially outward movement with the 'U'. In the pronunciation of 'U' the attempt to characterize something moving predominates. Thus with the eurythmical 'U' the physiologic opposite occurs: the ability to stand firm is called forth. This is present in the 'U' in artistic eurythmy as well, at least as a suggestion.

If you now take a look at the other vowels you will find a progressive internalization. In the case of the 'O' you have the lips pushed together towards the front and the opening of the mouth reduced in size—there is at least an attempt to reduce the size. This is transformed into the polar opposite in the encompassing gesture of the 'O'-movement in eurythmy. Precisely in such things the natural connections are to be perceived. In the manner in which 'O' is employed in speech certain forces are present. And in languages in which 'O' predominates one will find that the people have the greatest propensity to become obese. That may really be taken as a guideline for the study of the physiologic processes connected with speech. If one were to develop a language consisting principally of modifications of 'O', where people had to carry out the characteristic mouth and lip formation of the 'O' continuously, they would all become pot-bellied. If with the 'O', on the one hand, one has this propensity to become pot-bellied, as I would like to call it, it is easy to understand why when reversed the 'O' represents on the other hand that which combats this obesity when it is carried out eurythmically and in the metamorphosis demonstrated yesterday.

The state of affairs is different, for example, with 'E'. A language that is rich in 'E' will engender skinny people, weaklings. And that is related to what I said yesterday about the treatment of thin people, and thus of weaklings, in relation to the significance of 'E'. You will remember that I said that in the case of weaklings particularly the 'E'-movement with its given modification is to be applied.

Now in respect to all these matters, it is necessary, however, to take one thing into account. If we consider the forms outwardly we do not come to the truth of the matter; we must grasp them inwardly in the process of their becoming. We must concentrate less on what comes to outward expression and more on the tendency involved. The tendency to become fat can be combated by means of the 'O' and the tendency to remain thin by the 'E'. Attention must be drawn to these matters because when eurythmy is used for therapeutic purposes it is necessary to take more into consideration the forces that are present in the upper man tending to a

widening, and the forces present in the lower man tending to
the linear. So I have to say, that when man utters the 'O' he
actually broadens the living element.*

You see, when I draw it roughly, the head of man[22] is in a
way a sphere. Speaking spiritually-scientifically, it is a proper
reproduction of the earth sphere. It is a copy of all those
forces that are centralized in the sphere of the earth; it is
developed by what lies in the forces of the moon. This latter
builds it up in such a manner that it becomes a sort of earth
sphere. Of course, this is all actually connected with cos-
mology and cosmogeny. As the earth phase proceeded out of
the Moon phase,[23] so out of the forces that are so powerfully
at work in building up the human head—which of itself, of
course, intends to become a sphere and is modified only by
the chest and the other part of the body, being attached to it,
altering the spherical form—so, out of the moon-building
forces the head is formed. Left to itself, the head would
become a proper sphere. That is not the case, because the
other two parts of the human organism are connected with
the head and influence its shape.

When we pronounce the 'O', we try to express what is
expressed in its spherical form in the entire etheric head. One
makes the effort to form a second head for oneself [see the

---

* For the last phrase, the shorthand report is unclear: *weitet* could be read
as *bildet*; *das Lebendige* as *das Folgende*. This translates: 'he actually forms
what follows'.

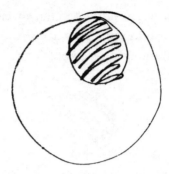

outer line of the circle in the drawing]. One can really say that, in uttering the 'O', man puffs himself up like his head— he puffs himself up, he blows himself out, awakening thereby the forces at the other pole that give him the tendency to become fat. These things can really be taken pictorially as well. The inflating of his own head gives him the tendency to become fat. When one wants to counteract this tendency to become, etherically-speaking, a fathead—not really a fathead, but etherically a fathead—to become a big head, then one must attempt to round it off from the other side, to take it back into oneself. And that is the protest of the fathead. Consequently an 'O' is formed as the opposite pole. All the individual sounds have a nuance of feeling, which is deeply established in the organism because it lies in the unconscious; hence the import of the inner essence of the sound. For the person who looks at the matter in a supersensory manner, the frog who would like to blow himself up into an ox [in the Grimms' story], you see, is the one from whom a cannon-like 'O'-sound would continuously proceed if he were able to fulfil his intention. That is the peculiarity of it— we have to explain by means of such things, if we want to understand these matters inwardly.

With the 'E' it is distinctly the reverse. In 'E' one wants to take hold of oneself inwardly, wants to contract together inwardly. For that reason there is the touching of oneself in eurythmy, this becoming aware of oneself. You become aware of yourself, simply, when you place the right arm upon the left, just as when you feel an object outside yourself. When you take a hold of it, you become aware of yourself. It would be even more clearly expressed if you simply grasped the right arm with the left hand (in art only an indication of all these things can be given), when you grasp the right arm with the left hand you are feeling yourself. This contacting oneself has come to expression especially in the eurythmical 'E'. And this touching oneself is carried out throughout the whole human organism. You can study this touching of yourself simply by studying the relationship of the nerve-process in the human back, those that ordinary physiology mistakenly call the motor nerves and those that are called sensory.

Here where the motor nerve, which is basically a sensory nerve too, comes together with the sensory nerve, a similar sort of clasping occurs. The fact is that the nerve-strands on the human back continually form an 'E'. In this forming of the 'E' lies the way in which man's inward perception of himself, which is factually differentiated, in the brain, comes into being. Yesterday we attempted to reproduce this 'E'-forming which actually takes place in a plane; you will find that what we attempted to reproduce shows, through the outward movement and the position of the movement, how this inward 'E'-forming in man is summed up in the vertical axis. As the head puffs itself out and wants to become a horn-blowing cherub, this 'E'-process, this pulling oneself together into a point, sums itself up in the vertical, in the perpendicular. It is a continuous and successive fastening together of 'E's which stand one above another; that expresses clearly what one observes taking place in weaklings. They have the tendency continuously to stretch their etheric bodies. They want to extend the etheric body rather than to pull it together into a point, which would be the real antithesis to the activity of the head. That is not, however, the case. They try to stretch the etheric body, thereby making a repetition of the point. And this extension which makes its appearance in people who are becoming weak—not the stretching in the physical, but the stretching in the etheric body—will be counteracted by shaping that 'E', of which we spoke yesterday.

So, I believe, you will see now how there is an inward connection between the eurythmical element involved and the human formative tendencies, how what is present in him as formative tendencies has been drawn out of the human being. The fact is that these formative tendencies, expressing themselves first in growth, in the forming of man, in his configuration, become specialized and localized once again in the development of the speech organism, this special organism. There these formative tendencies—which are otherwise spread out over the entire person—are to an extent accumulated. In developing eurythmy we now return. We proceed from the localized tendency to the whole man, thus placing another specialization in opposition to the specialization of the human organization in the speech organism, the specialization in the will-organism. The whole human being is indeed an expression of his volitional nature, in so far as he is throughout metabolic and limb organism. One can move this or that part of the head, too, and consequently the head is also in a certain sense limb-organism. That can be demonstrated by those people who are capable in this respect of a little more than others. People who can wiggle their ears, and so on, they can show very clearly how the principle of movement of the limbs, the limb-nature, extends into the organization of the head. The whole human being is in this respect an expression of the volitional nature. When we go on to eurythmy, we express this volition once again. Before we proceed tomorrow to work out the sounds specifically, to the special manner of forming them, and further to the combinations of sounds, I would like to speak in closing of something historical.

The movement of the will and the movement of the intellect, you see, constitute two sorts of evolution of power which proceed in man at different velocities. Man's intellect develops quickly in our age, volition slowly, so that as part of the whole evolution of mankind we have already surpassed our will with our intellect. In our civilization it is generally manifest that the evolution of the intellect has overtaken the evolution of the will. The people of today are intensely intellectual, which precisely does *not* imply that they can do much with their intellect. They are strongly intellectual, but they hardly know what to do with their intellect; for this reason they know so little intellectually. But what they do know intellectually they treat in such a manner as though within it they could function with certainty. Will develops slowly. And to practise eurythmy is, apart from everything else, an attempt to bring the will back into the whole evolution of humankind again. If eurythmy is to appear as a therapy the following must be pointed out. It must be said that the overdevelopment of the intellect expresses itself particularly in the organic side-effects of the evolution of speech as well. Our speech-development today in our modern civilization is actually already something which is becoming inhuman through its superhuman qualities—in so far as we learn languages today in such a manner that we have so little living feeling left for what lies in the words. The words are actually only signs. What sort of feeling do people still command for what lies in words? I would like to know how many people go through the world and become aware in the course, for example, of learning the German language, that the rounded form which I have just drawn is expressed in the word *Kopf*, 'head', which has a connection with *Kohl*, 'cabbage'. For which reason one also says *Kohlkopf*, 'cabbage-head', which is actually only a repetition; the rounding is metamorphosed according to the situation. That is what is expressed here. In the Romance languages, *testa*, *testieren*, expresses more what comes from within, the working of the soul through the head. People have no more feeling for the distinctions within language; language has become abstract. When you walk, you walk with your feet. Why do we say *Fusse*, 'feet'? You see, that is a metamorphosis of the word *Furche*, 'furrow', which came about because it was seen that one traces something like a furrow when one walks. The pictorial element in language has been completely lost. If one wishes to bring this pictorial element back into language, then one must turn to eurythmy.

Every word that is experienced non-pictorially is actually an inward cause of illness; I am speaking with coarse words now—but then we only have coarse words—of something which expresses itself in the finer human organism. Civilized humankind suffers chronically today from the effects which learning to speak abstractly, which the failure to experience words pictorially, has upon it. The results are so far-reaching that, in those people who have made their language abstract, the accompanying organic side-effects express themselves as a very strong tendency towards irregularities in the rhythmic system and a refusal to function of the metabolic system. However, we can actually do something about what is being spoilt in people today through language, which is acquired of course in early childhood. If it is acquired in a non-pictorial way, it really produces conditions leading later on to all kinds of illnesses. We can actually fight against this with the help of therapeutic eurythmy. Eurythmy therapy may be introduced in a thoroughly organic manner into therapeutic treatment as a whole.

It is truly so; the person who understands that developing oneself spiritually has always something to do with becoming ill—this must be taken into account in the course of spiritual development—must also take into consideration that one can fight this process of becoming ill which is due to our civilization, not alone with outward physical studies [*Studien*], but also with outward methods/remedies [*Mitteln*]. We put soul and spirit into the movements of eurythmy and combat thereby what, on the other side, soul and spirit do themselves, though often in earliest childhood, in such a manner that the effect of their activity when it develops in later life is felt to be the cause of illness. That is what I wanted to say today.

Lecture 4

Dornach, 15 April 1921

My dear friends, as we have seen, the vowels in eurythmy always work more or less directly on the rhythmic organism. With the consonantal eurythmical movements the case is that, although the rhythmic organism is, of course, also affected, this is accomplished by way of the system of the metabolism and limbs. Naturally, the first thing we have to do today is simply to take a look at the details; here one can arrive at a contemplative picture of what is involved only when one can enter into the details.

We will now go through the most important consonantal movements in eurythmy. Perhaps you would do a 'B' for us, Frl. Wolfram; and now this 'B' in walking as well. Try to walk in such a manner, however, that one leg imitates the motion of the arm while moving; but repeat the 'B'. Now imagine that done ever more quickly and repeated, initially, let's say, for four to five minutes. Perhaps Fr. Baumann will now do the 'P' for us in the same manner. The difference is not very great. Now attempt to do this with the legs as well. That brings about a complicated leg movement which is very similar to the movements of music eurythmy (not stepping down in between). That must now be repeated frequently and in series by the person with whom you hope to accomplish something by means of the 'P'. Now, all the movements that are connected with the eurythmical consonants have to do with that which, in the process of digestion, lies on the other side (*jenseits*) of the activity of the stomach and intestine. We will now ignore the actual intestinal space through which the food passes. When we consider the outer wall of the intestine, however, where the chyme passes through the intestinal villi, and so on, and then into the blood and the lymph—thus from the other side of that comprised in the first digestive activity—the movement such as we have just made works back on the inward digestion, on all that is digestive activity in the blood vessels, and in particular on what is digestive activity in the kidneys. If you are concerned with regulating the activity of the kidneys, you should have such movements carried out. Precisely the movements that we have just done, 'B' and 'P', are those that work pre-eminently in the regulation of renal activity, for example, in regulating the elimination of urine. These connections are certainly extraordinarily interesting for someone who recalls how the whole circulatory being of man is related to language, and how a connection arises between that which pushes itself into the circulatory system from the metabolic system and this particular manner of making sounds, of making consonants.

Let us try to carry out a 'D'. Now attempt to do the same movement with the legs. You hop, and while hopping you bend the legs somewhat at the knee. Here, try to get the patients to bend at the knees and hop, bending ever more strongly, and have them jump. Perhaps Frau Baumann will demonstrate the 'T' for us; here the corresponding movement will be a hop forwards with an attempt at making knock-knees (*X-Beine*, 'X-legs'). While stepping forward you make the attempt to hop forwards and outwards and form knock-knees. That is what is to be carried out. Our first concern is to demonstrate these things. So we have 'D' and 'T'. When one carries out what we call the soft sound, one can remedy milder conditions; with what we call the hard sound, the more severe conditions of this sort. These sounds 'D' and 'T' are really like this. Of course, you must have the patients repeat them for several minutes until they are quite tired—in these things it is really a matter of carrying the exercise out until one is tired. And when one carries them out to fatigue, the sounds 'D' and 'T' in particular are a force which works to strengthen the intestinal activity, particularly when that activity manifests itself in constipation. In this manner one can counteract constipation in many cases. Such a matter is unquestionably evident to the person who knows the physiological connections between the speech organism which takes up the movement in the course of learning to speak, and the system of the metabolism and limbs.

Now perhaps you will be so good, Frl. Wolfram, and demonstrate the 'G'-sound for us. Here it is a matter of trying again to hop forwards in a similar manner while forming knock-knees. It would be the same thing with the 'K'-sound (Frau Baumann). And now you must try to move forwards with the legs spread out sharply, with the 'Q' as well; but that is the same thing. Here in the case of 'G', as well as of 'K' and of 'Q', we have a movement which stimulates the forward motion, the inner mechanization of the intestine, which thus promotes the movement of the intestine itself. The difference in the physiological effect of 'D' and 'T', 'G', 'K', and 'Q', is that in the case of 'D' and 'T' the processing of the food itself is more affected, while with 'G', 'K', and 'Q' the effect is more on the forward motion of the food in the intestine when the intestine itself lags. Particularly important and therapeutically fruitful is the 'S'. When you do the 'S'-sound it is necessary to hop, to hop forwards keeping the legs continuously in the 'O'-form, and to do the 'S'-sound. Because one continually sets the legs down in this 'O'-shape, this actually has a very inward connection with the human digestive activity, and that is with the metabolic activity as it works back upon the entire human organism. In this movement we have something which we can have those children do who show an insufficent digestive activity and who consequently have headaches, since this movement regulates in particular the formation of gas in the intestine. When this is not in order, when it is either insufficient or too strong, this movement in particular will have a most important effect.

Then we have the 'F'-sound (Frau Baumann). We have to do here with something of a soul-nature. Try to perform the jump in the following manner. You begin and try to go forwards; in landing you must come down strictly on the tips of the toes, however, and now bring the heels down—once again, a jump onto the tips of the toes, then down onto the heels again. In the case of the 'V', it would be just the same. Here we have a movement which should be practised when you find that urination is not in order. It has a stimulating effect on the passing of urine. When it is necessary to stimulate this—for whatever reason—here is the movement to be performed.

It is, of course, entirely possible to combine the movements in the most varied manners; you will find in giving treatment that you will have to combine the one with the other, depending on the direction to be taken.

If we do an 'R' (Frl. Wolfram), I must ask you please to do it in such a way that in stepping forwards you always stretch distinctly, then with the left foot thus [here the lecturer demonstrated the bending and stretching movement himself], put the weight on the foot, stretch and as you step forwards—continuing in this manner to step on the foot with the legs bent—try to do the 'R'. That would have to be developed in this manner. If this 'R' is practised with a person for a few minutes, one would have to practise it frequently during the day, however—then it is something which regulates the rhythm of evacuation if that is not in order. That is something which works directly over onto the rhythm of evacuation and regulates it.

In observing the whole dynamics of the human being, it will be important to keep in view the connections which come to light arising out of the diagnosis, and do these movements not in a dilettante fashion but in a manner suitable to the matter at hand.

Now an 'L' (Fr. Baumann); here again together with the effort to place the legs in the knock-kneed position and hop forwards, draw together, now once again. It should be an effort to hop forwards, too! The forwards motion is absolutely necessary in such a case. This movement works especially strongly on the peristalsis, on the movement of the intestine itself. With this movement you can also have the patient move backwards in the same manner. He/she will experience much more difficulty in learning to do it. But it will have a significant effect in regulating the movement of the intestine itself, the peristalsis, as all these movements in fact work in a regulative manner out of the system of the limbs and the metabolism into what in this context is a dependency of the system of limbs and metabolism (or at least adjacent to it), that is, into the circulation and into the respiratory movement as well.

A very interesting letter is the 'H', which actually is attached to most vowels. Accompany the 'H' in walking as follows: try to stand with the legs together, to hop forwards, and in the course of this hop forwards to spread the legs and strike the floor with the legs apart; you should always be moving forwards. That is a movement which, I beg you to take notice, must be carried out absolutely slowly. In the case of the other movements it is important to carry them out quickly; this movement, however, is to be carried out slowly and there must be pauses for rest between each of the jumps as well. This must be taken into account with this movement, as it has a very strong effect on the regulation of intestinal activity in the area of transition from the stomach into the intestine. So, when you notice that someone cannot get his food from the stomach into the intestine, it will be greatly to his advantage to perform this movement, but, as I said, tranquilly and standing still after each separate hop.

Now we have the 'M' (Fr. Baumann). This 'M' is to be made with the *Kibitz*, 'peewit-step'. It is good to do one step with one leg and the next with the other leg—forwards and back. One can also do the peewit-step backwards and then with the other leg forwards again. This technique of doing the peewit-step backwards is something which one should really master. It is in fact a movement which it is important to study, for when the 'M' is carried out in this form in move-ment it acts to regulate the entire system of the metabolism and the limbs. It is extraordinarily important to practise it with the children during puberty. When this exercise with 'M' is practised at the time of sexual maturity it will prove a strong regulator of over-assertive sexuality. It will regulate over-assertive sexuality when practised during puberty. You must only have developed an eye for whether it should be practised in this manner. It is not without reason that the 'M' was regarded as an especially important sound in the time when people still understood something of the inner content of the sounds; it is the sound which closes the 'OM'-syllable of the East. The 'OM'-syllable of the East is closed by 'M' because the whole human being is in fact regulated through the system of the metabolism and the limbs by precisely this sound. So this movement is particularly regulatory. In early cultures it was absolutely customary to have the younger people perform such movements in order to educate them to be corporally complete human beings and, at the same time, human beings exercising self-control.

Then we have the 'N'-sound. The 'N'-sound is accompanied by a jump in which the knees are bent from the beginning. So, one keeps the legs, the knees, bent and then jumps. That is a movement which greatly strengthens the intestinal activity, and in such a manner that it can be applied where there is a tendency to diarrhoea. That can serve as a substantiation or as an indication of how one can see the effect of the system of movement on the metabolic system. That is something which you really only notice when you consider the connections between the system of movement and the metabolic system in the light of your knowledge of the threefold arrangement of the human organism. This threefold ordering of the human organism in fact sheds light on many things; in our present time where knowledge of the soul consists almost solely of words, one can think out at length all sorts of exercises in which one believes one has taken the soul-element into account—or one can develop gymnastics in which one takes only the bodily physiology into consideration. One can talk round about at length on these matters; without knowledge of the threefold ordering of the human organism one will not attain any clarity. It was interesting, in fact, to have a physiologist of the present day[24] here who listened to one of the introductions that I usually give at eurythmy performances, and then saw eurythmy as well. Now, I normally say that in education one will have to replace the sort of gymnastics that proceeds solely from physiology with this soul-filled sort of gymnastics.[25] Thereupon the physiologist, who is also known as a very great authority in nutritional matters, said that for him it wasn't enough to say that one shouldn't overrate gymnastics; for him gymnastics was no method of education at all, but a barbarism.

Now, you see, behind something like this is hidden a very important symptom of the times. It is, on the one hand, just as correct to say that the gymnastics of today is usually one-sidedly conceived—since it is taken out of the physiology and anatomy of the organism alone—as it is at least one-sided on the other hand to say that gymnastics is a barbarism. Why? Because when one develops gymnastics out of the physiology of the body alone it does become a barbarism. It is our materialistic education and civilization that first made a barbarism out of gymnastics. In the manner in which gymnastics is practised today, it is a barbarism. And this conception of gymnastics is connected with some completely false notions, is it not? For example, people believe—although the experts don't believe it any more, still many people believe—that if one has a person exert himself mentally and then allows him to recover, as they believe, in body afterwards, that constitutes a proper recuperation. But that isn't true at all! If a person does arithmetic or gymnastics for an hour he will become equally tired in reality; it makes no difference. That is known today, but people cannot properly judge how soul and spirit should be brought into gymnastic movements, how the movements carried out are to proceed from the human being as a whole. Gymnastics will have to be developed gradually, in such a way that what we are developing as artistic eurythmy can unite with what is developed as physiological gymnastics. One can make the transition from the eurythmical to the gymnastic quite well. It will only be necessary to see that this sort of eurythmy, which actually takes the part of a kind of soul-filled gymnastics in the lesson, is done with humour; above all it must be enjoyable for the children. It must give the children joy; that belongs to it. To teach eurythmy like a grumpy, dried-out schoolmaster would be something which could really not be done at all!

Now we still have the 'Sh' (Frl. Wolfram). When it is accompanied by a small jump, then a larger jump; a small jump, then again a larger jump; a smaller jump, a larger jump, then one has a movement with a strong effect in the 'Sh' as well; however, it too must be carried out slowly. It is not necessary to slow the 'N'-movement down particularly, but with the 'H'-movement ['M' in the original stenogram was corrected to 'H' in pencil] and the 'Sh'-movement it is essential to do them slowly, and in the case of the latter to take a short rest after every three jumps, at the transition to the next series. In this way a rhythm is brought into it as well: short, long, short—and now one rests—long, short, long—and now a rest—short, long, short—now a rest. One has in this movement, which in the appropriate cases—one can combine movements, of course—affects the beginning portions of the intestinal tract that pertains to the stomach. When someone has what is in itself such a weak digestion that the food remains lying in the stomach (I have drawn attention to similar matters on other occasions), that will also be particularly the case where the 'H'-movement is involved. With the 'Sh'-movement, however, you have to notice, for example, whether stomach acidity easily occurs and so on; then the 'Sh'-movement should be carried out.

So you see, the consonants as they are done eurythmically

are connected with the formation of man in a totally different manner from the eurythmical vowels. When we considered the doing of vowels in eurythmy, I had to draw your attention to the manner in which the inward, that which lies more to the interior, is related to movement. Here we have to do with the effect on the third member of the threefold organism.

When applying what we discussed the day before yesterday in regard to the vowels, it would be good to have the patient sound the vowel of the exercise to be done, slowly, before the exercise as such is begun. So, without singing—singing would be of less help in this case—he very simply intones the sound at length, 'A', 'I', and when he has done this for a time, when he has sounded it out loud, you would have him carry out the movement for the vowel in question. When he has done that, you should try to call forth in him the impression that he hears the sound that he has just carried out, as if he heard it. You will find that in the present day only very few people have the mental picture that they hear the sounds inwardly in a soul-and-spirit manner. So we have to tell him to enter into a state of soul such as if he were to hear the 'I' (*ee*). It is particularly important to understand this matter. Then, you see, when you have the patient speak the vowel, intone it, the organism as such feels as if the sound were being induced. If he then carries out the movement, it appears to be the result of the spoken sound. And then one listens. One intones the 'I', then does the movement that we have learnt, and then in one's imagination imagines that one hears the 'I' sounding. Then we have: the calling forth of the 'I', that which arises through the movement of the 'I', the hearing of that which has moved, and the hearing of the sound once again. This is something which brings a great deal of life into this human etheric body; and in precisely those directions we have pointed out, it brings real life into the etheric body. In these matters, in these exercises the intention is to bring movement into the human etheric body, to bring an inwardly regulated movement into the etheric activity of the human organism. It is particularly interesting to see how the movement, which as a movement of the intestine progresses from the front to the back, releases a movement in the etheric body which proceeds from back to front and then breaks on the abdominal wall—it does not actually 'break', but disappears. This latter movement is in most cases where the intestinal activity is not in order, in gross disorder as well. This activity which counters the physical movement will be aroused, for example, particularly by the 'R'-movement. Here there is a very lively vibrating from back to front; that is the element in the 'R'-movement which affects the rhythm of evacuation in a very specific manner.

It can also be used educationally as the whole human organism is a unity and everything in it works together. If you were to survey children in school, for example, you would find amongst them some who can hardly pronounce an 'R', who are quite shocking in their pronunciation of the 'R'. Of course, other factors can play in and the matter may not be self-evident—nevertheless, such children are always simul-taneously candidates for becoming hardened physically (*Hartleibigkeit*). One does them a service, in fact, by doing something with them such as I showed you yesterday—the 'R'-movement, which affects the rhythm of evacuation positively. It is indeed possible to make use of these things in education. Here you only need to indicate; you must not go too far. The physician, however, can go much further as he will find that specific symptoms naturally appear when the exercise is practised for days and weeks. But he is, of course in the position by other means to counter these symptoms, which quite justifiably appear. I want to point out that if the effect of the 'N'-movement [in the stenogram clearly 'M' and in earlier editions 'N'—a mistake in what was heard?] were to become too predominant, you would only have to counteract it with the 'D'-movement and you would nevertheless have achieved what was to be achieved. One can balance the one by means of the other.

The only other thing I wish to say today is that I really do not want artistic eurythmy to be influenced in any way whatsoever by the discussion which must of course arise when eurythmy is considered as a discipline for health and therapy. I beg the artistic eurythmists to forget these things thoroughly when they practise artistic eurythmy, so that they are not confused by their thoughts on digestive activity when they are involved in artistic eurythmy. That would be most disconcerting! One must nevertheless be entirely clear that human art does have to do with the whole human being; it does not proceed from the head alone. That must naturally be kept in view especially in the case of an art of movement. That is what I wanted to tell you today. In the following days, we will discuss more what has to do with human evolution, with reference to what comes to the fore after certain intervals of time, that is to say, what occurs at a later age, as the consequence of an exercise affecting the organism of the child.

Lecture 5

Dornach, 16 April 1921

My dear friends, today we will turn to some of those eurythmical exercises more related to the activity proceeding from the soul. Before we begin, however, it will be necessary to take note that it is usually assumed when a person produces an expression of will or when he arrives at a judgement that these expressions are connected with the human nervous system alone. This, however, is not at all the case. One must make it clear to oneself that the judgements which the human being passes, for example, are bound up with his entire constitution, that man pronounces a judgement out of the totality of his being.[26] So, when you do the eurythmical movement corresponding to a judgement, here again, the whole human being is influenced in a certain manner; it is not only the head which will be subject to the influences of what arises through judging eurythmically. Frau Baumann will show us the movement that corresponds to affirmation, and then the one corresponding to negation. Naturally, when used as a therapeutic exercise it should be carried out several times without interruption. This affirmation and negation is precisely what can be called a judgement in the general sense; when one confirms or negates something one has to do with the nature of judgement in its essence. When you give such an affirmation or negation, the movement, when it is repeated frequently, works very strongly on the respiratory system by way of a detour through the etheric body. By this means you can counter a tendency to shortness of breath.

You can repeat the affirmation, for example, ten times consecutively, then the negation, and follow this up with affirmation—negation, affirmation—negation, both ten times consecutively. Of whatever illness this shortness of breath may be the symptom, by this means you will be able to counteract it in such a way that the entire constitution is affected, as the whole matter occurs by way of a detour through the etheric body. You only have to keep in view what is being done here. We might interpret what Frau Baumann has done, touching upon what is essential in it, as follows. What she thereby projects into the world is a thought that has become fleeting, a thought that has gained wings and gone over into movement. When a judgement is fixed eurythmically—as an affirmation or negation—then it is a thought which rides on the movement. And because the thought rides on the movement, on the one hand you in fact project outwards a part of this being; on the other hand, because the thought rides on the movement you take a part more thoroughly into yourself than otherwise. That is to say, you do a movement through which you become more awake than you otherwise are. Such movements are actually movements that awaken. However, because you do not wake up with the 'I', the ego, at the same time in the same manner, the activity of the ego is in a certain way dampened. This dampening of the ego-activity, though, is not absolute, but [occurs] in relation to the organism. In fighting shortness of breath by means of this detour through the etheric body, this constitutes what would be the first symptom reached and what is introduced into the whole human constitution by means of the byway through the etheric body.

Now, a disposition of the will—sympathy and antipathy. [Frl. Wolfram demonstrates.] Imagine you do this movement repeatedly, one after another: sympathy—antipathy, sympathy—antipathy, or only one of these two. When you do this, in a certain sense you are setting out something which you carry within yourself; naturally this can only be confirmed through observation. It is a kind of falling asleep. The other movement [affirmation and negation] must be carried out quickly; this must be carried out slowly. It is indeed a movement which brings forth the imagination of sleep in the observer; imaginatively you fall asleep with such a movement—not in reality, however, at least that shouldn't happen! But because in reality you don't fall asleep while making this movement, the 'I' is more strongly active in relation to the body than it usually is. By means of such a movement the circulation and the digestion as a whole are stimulated. The entire digestion is really stimulated in such a manner that through such a movement the tendency to belch, for example, can be counteracted.

Now we want to express what we could call 'the feeling of love[27] towards something' (Frau Baumann will demonstrate). Take a good look at this, the feeling of love for something. Imagine it carried out ten times consecutively and accompanied by a powerful 'E' between each of the movements. Thus, Love—'E', Love—'E', and so on, one after another. You accompany the movements which you have learned as expressing feeling in eurythmy—it could be another feeling as well—with the movement for 'E'. Here we have a strong influence which proceeds from the human etheric acting on the astral nature, and which has the effect of warming the circulation. It is something which really works on the circulatory system in a beneficial manner. One cannot say that it accelerates or retards the circulation; it affects it in a beneficially warming manner.

We also have something which could be called a wish: hope (Frl. Wolfram). Look at this and picture to yourself that you repeatedly carry out this movement for the wish—always returning to the position of balance, then carrying out the movement for the wish again—and always alternating it with the movement for 'U'. This means that the astral will act very strongly upon the etheric nature, and it can be said that a beneficial warming effect on the breathing system will result. Naturally, you have to take into consideration that all these things of which we have spoken today occur by way of a detour through the etheric body, and consequently never show what effect they have on the following day. Some effects may appear after two to three days, yet then they are all the more certain.

Now imagine that we do a bending and stretching movement with the legs and at the same time a definite 'B'-movement (Frau Baumann). That which I have just shown you simultaneous with a decided 'B'-movement, now rest, 'B' while bending, ten times consecutively. Then pause and again ten times. This is something which people should do who very frequently suffer from migraine or other head-aches.[28] The time for them to do it, however, is not when they are suffering from the headache, but rather when they are not.

A particularly effective movement is the following. Bend and stretch the torso forwards and backwards, accompanying this movement simultaneously with the movement for 'R' [Frl. Wolfram]. Bend forwards, bend backwards with the 'R'; that consecutively and often. This positively affects the whole rhythmic system, the rhythm of breathing and of the circulation. When there are irregularities present there, this will work extraordinarily well under all conditions.

Now I will ask you to take a look at another most effective movement which consists in shaking the head to the right and left with the movement for 'M'. The head should not be turned, as far as possible, but only bent to the right and left, and that with the 'M'-movement. This is something which when practised has a very strong quieting effect on all possible irregularities in the lower body, again by way of a detour through the etheric body. Irregularities in the lower system, expressing themselves through pains, can thereby be mitigated. You have to combat tendencies to such pains when the pains are *not* present. That is the crux of the matter. While the pains are present, it cannot very well be carried out. The important thing is to carry it out as long as the pains are not present.

Please take note of the following. Press against* the knee with the other foot, and accompany this with an 'E'-movement of the arms. This bending of one leg, hitting the other leg, is accompanied by an 'E'-movement of the arms. It is a very beautiful movement. It can and should be carried out as an exercise with children in school, for carried out frequently it treats the most varied aspects of clumsiness.[29] The children will at least be well cured of their clumsiness when they practise just this exercise. And when the children come and say that their shoulders hurt so and everything possible hurts, then you reply, 'That is exactly what I wanted; you will be especially glad about it once it's better again!' Every pain that is brought about in this manner combats clumsiness. With respect to this, one can deal quite energetically with the children.

---

* The word *schlagen*, 'strike', is found in H. Finckh's transcript, but is unreadable in her shorthand report.

Now we will take a look at another variation [of movement]. Imagine every sort of 'E'-movement that can be carried out with the arms now projected onto the floor. This movement comes into existence when this line crosses the other diagonally.* Now let us imagine it in this way. Frau Baumann places herself here, Frl. Wolfram there. Now walk and accompany the whole thing with an 'E'-movement with the arms. Move so that you pass by one another, but pay attention that you don't run into each other. So you do an 'E' on the floor and an 'E' with the arms, paying attention at the same time that you don't collide. It is this taking notice of the other person, this exerting of your concentration on him/her combined with the 'E'-gesture, which works together here with the movement. This exercise can only be carried out with two people. When carried out by two people, it is essentially what we would call a strengthening of the heart, all that which is connected with the phenomena which we generally term the strengthening of the heart.

Question: Could one have this exercise carried out by one sick and one healthy person? You can readily do that, but you would perhaps have to have the healthy person omit the 'E'-movement with the arms. This movement is especially intended for the clinical situation where one will, of course, have two people in need of a strengthening of the heart; it really is better if you have two such people.

Now let us imagine the movement like this. One of the ladies stands here, the other here, behind one another. When you [Fr. Baumann] arrive here, then Frl. Wolfram carries out

---

* A sketch, which appeared in earlier editions, is to be found neither in the shorthand report nor in the transcript; it is not reproduced in the German 5th edition.

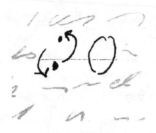

the path which you have begun, but in such a manner that she is always facing forwards. Then as the movement carries on, you take this part of the path and you the other. You initiate the continuation of your own movement in the other person, accompanying it with the 'O'-position of the arms. Now, you will see that the people who do this begin at a certain tempo; to begin with it must be slower, then become ever faster and faster. This rapid tempo should then ebb out into a slower one. That is a movement which serves significantly to strengthen the diaphragm, and thereby the whole breathing system. Here again, if you leave out the 'O'-movement with the arms you can have a healthy person participate, but it is of course best to employ two people who are in need of therapy.

Now I will ask you, Frau Baumann, to demonstrate the 'H'-movement for us once again. This is an 'H'-movement. I will ask you to do this movement in such a way that you hold the arms still and imitate the movement with the shoulders alone as well as possible. In this case, however, one must accustom oneself to doing this movement with the shoulders, making an 'A' with the arms at the same time, an 'A' of any sort with the arms. That should be repeated frequently. You see, that is what could be designated as 'laughing eurythmically'. That is how one laughs eurythmically. When one laughs thus eurythmically that which one has in the therapeutic effect of laughing itself[30] is really very greatly heightened. The therapeutic effect of laughing is well known. But when one practises laughing eurythmically, this therapeutic effect is proportionately greater. But you could do it otherwise as well.

Frl. Wolfram, please do an 'A'-movement of some sort. And now try to do the same movement I spoke of before, the shoulder movement of the 'H', but do it quite slowly as if you wished to do it thoughtfully. Thus into the 'A'-movement of the arms you do the shoulder movement of the 'H'. We could designate that as follows. The whole organism is brought into accord with the feeling of veneration. It encompasses all that which the feeling of veneration actually effects in the organism. The effect on the human organism of the feeling of veneration, when it is habitual, is to make the organism as such actually more durable, more sturdy. It becomes capable of greater resistance. People who really have the capacity for veneration inherent in them become more capable of resistance within their organism. That is why everything which brings children to veneration, to the gift or capacity for reverence,[31] makes children more resilient. You can come to the assistance of this capacity for resilience through this last-described eurythmical exercise.

Keep in mind that what we have demonstrated today as decision, expression of will, hope, love, what we have shown in respect to certain organic pains, what we have demonstrated as a means of combating clumsiness, and so on, all these things are related to man in such a way that the human being is gripped through them in the innermost part of his organic being and, by way of a detour through the etheric body, actually gives the possibility of making this etheric body into a workable instrument. The etheric body is a part of man which becomes stiff in most of those people who sit out their lives, spend their lives without interest for their surroundings. It is not good when the human etheric body becomes stiff, neither for the organic functions is it good. When you have the exercises which we have described today carried out by children in moderation, and by the appropriate patients very energetically (one can see by the indications given which patients have need of them), the etheric body will become supple and inwardly flexible.[32] And by means of them you will do the children as well as the adults a good service.

These movements are indeed such that one can give them priority over the usual gymnastic movements;[33] the usual gymnastic movements are taken in reality from the physiology, from the *physis* of the body alone, and they tear the physical body continually out of the etheric body. The physical body then does its own movements which do *not* pull after them the movements of the etheric body in the corresponding manner. For this reason the usual, merely physiological gymnastics is basically a school for materialism, since by means of it materialistic thought is transformed into feeling. Eurythmy makes man more capable of recognizing himself within himself, of gaining inner control over himself. Consequently, such exercises have an educational, instructive value as well as a therapeutic and healthy value. The attempt should be made to have these exercises—those described today, I mean—carried out in moderation also by adults and to develop them in such a way that they could be carried out by the sick in a clinical situation.

A question has been put to me which could perhaps lead to something—and some other questions as well. Here is the question: 'The Chinese cannot pronounce the letter R, they substitute L for it. "Strawberries", for example, become "stlawbellies". Does that have to do with their race?'

It has to do, of course, with the organization of the organism, in so far as that is racially determined. Through the particular gift of one part of mankind for one sound or another, we can see what tendencies are inherent in certain people by virtue of their race. I brought such things to discussion just a few sessions ago.[34]

Other questions have been put about exercises which could be used in relation to conditions of indolence, insufficient reaction, lethargy, and so on—conditions which frequently have to do with an insufficient thyroid activity. And here it has been brought to our attention that Fliess—in his well-known book[35] about the course of life—has placed this complex of symptoms in the intermediate sexual category. How could a contemporary author not do so? Everything about which he knows very little, he chalks up to the intermediate sexual category, or some other way. He puts, for example, gauche [*linkisch* = clumsy, left-handed] people in the same category.* I want expressly to emphasize, however, that I have never recommended a eurythmical exercise with a special right-left emphasis to anyone.

[*Attention was drawn to the exercises (from lecture 1), which should be begun either to the right or to the left: iambus, trochee.*]

It is not in order particularly to accentuate an emphasis on the right or left, but rather in order to call forth the feeling of the iambus or trochee within the forward-motion. That is thoroughly justified. The fact is that it has less to do with the

---

* In the shorthand report a fragmentary sentence appears, not transcribed by H. Finckh. It may have referred to diligence. See the references given in the notes.

long-short than it has to do with the particular movement. It is quite correct; it has to do with the fact that what lives in the breathing system is reversed when it is transferred into the system of movement. The upper man and the lower man are the reverse of one another. Thus every imaginable iambus in the breathing system, brought forth in speech, has of necessity to become a trochee in the movement of legs and vice versa. Eurythmy in its entirety is based on this principle. You may test the whole of eurythmy in respect to it—eurythmy does not follow the principle of similarity in its execution, but the movement which is in keeping with the polar image. It is all entirely in accord with the image formed as the other polarity. This idea must be maintained throughout. But I have never recommended to anyone that he do something especially right or left; that should be left completely to the feelings. The question of whether a thing should be done with the right hand or the left hand should be determined only by those matters which would otherwise come into consideration. I do not want people to gain the impression that I would have suggested an emphasis on the right in particular eurythmical exercises for any gauche [*linkisch*], left-sided person. That is not the case.

In addition to this, I would like to emphasize the following. It is the case that when one has to do with insufficient reaction or with lethargy this more general indication will fall into some category which I have already given; lethargy is a general expression and can be relegated to something or other about which I have spoken. The appropriate movements should then be carried out.

[*Here a posed question does not appear in the shorthand report.*]

This condition of indolence, of lethargy, inattention and so on, as far as laziness, is to a certain extent a preliminary to

what is called in homoeopathy a diffuse★ mental condition
[... *a long gap in the shorthand report*]. Now what this involves,
purely medically, I will answer tomorrow morning [with the
doctors]. But since the question does link to the lecture on
eurythmy, I would like to say that on the whole such an
exercise as I have given here in connection with judgement
and expression of will has to be seen, especially with the
appearance of indolence, of lethargy, that it can be combated
very especially by what I have given for the expression of will.
If you should notice that this is not particularly effective, you
can alternate that exercise with the exercise I have given for
judgement, but in such a way that you attempt to discover—
as it is here a question of trying it out—whether it is more
effective when you vary the expression of will and the
expression of judgement in a ratio of 3:2 or of 2:3, that is, the
one shorter, the other longer. And since these things work by
way of a detour through the etheric body, you will find that
you will first have to begin and carry on with these exercises
for two to three days; according to the circumstances—when
you see that they are not having the proper effect—make a
change on the third day. But in general we can say that the
one exercise as well as the other will have an awakening effect
on man in both directions. The will exercise and the judgement exercise are the ones that come into particular consideration.

In order that there be no misunderstanding, I emphasize
that of course the opinion must not arise that these exercises
would have a very significant effect after being carried out for

---

★ The shorthand reporter, H. Finckh, first wrote *diffusen*, but was unsure,
underlining it and marking it with a cross. The German text retains her
second entry: *typhösen Geisteszustand*—typhoid mental/spiritual condition.

two or three days. That would be an error. In order to produce an effect, these exercises should be carried out for at least seven weeks. One can maintain—without necessarily being mystically inclined—that the space of time necessary for the beneficial effects just described to show themselves would be about seven weeks.

That is what I wanted to tell you today concerning these matters. I would like to request that the corresponding session tomorrow follow the other directly, after a short pause. Tomorrow will be the last eurythmy session, as it will be necessary to have two purely medical sessions one after the other on Monday.[36]

Lecture 6

My dear friends, there is such an infinite amount one could relate about the connections between health, therapy and eurythmy. Today we want to take into consideration that part of the physiological element that we discover in the proximity of the spiritual element when we look at a eurythmical exercise. Of course, all that can be observed in this connection in artistic eurythmy will be encountered in an intensified form when we make the transition from artistic eurythmy to the fortified eurythmy we have become acquainted with in these days. Nevertheless, the essence of what concerns us can already be discovered when eurythmy is carried out purely artistically and the physiology corresponding to it can then be found. Let us try this by carrying out the following.

Perhaps Frau Baumann will be so good and perform the poem *Über allen Gipfeln ist Ruh*[37] alternately in vowels and in consonants, while you [Frau Dr Steiner][38] perhaps recite it.

Über allen Gipfeln ist Ruh'
In allen Wipfeln
Spürest Du
Kaum einen Hauch
Die Vögelein schweigen
Im Walde
Warte nur
Balde ruhest Du auch.

Now stillness covers
All the hill-tops
Hardly a breath stirs.
The birds are in the forest
Have finished their song.
Wait you too shall rest
Before long.
(Tr. David Luke)

Now let us make clear to ourselves what is taking place here, proceeding however very exactly. What is happening? A poem is recited. The person who does the eurythmy listens— he is the one who comes for us into consideration physiologically. That is the first matter of importance. He doesn't speak himself, he actively listens. That is essential. He actively listens to something that is in essence the meaningful word, a meaningful association of words.[39] He listens to something in which the activity of thought and of mental picturing is alive. What he perceives outwardly is the activity of mental picturing clothed in an association of sounds. That is something which man in his waking, daytime existence often does, is it not? But what actually takes place when in his waking, daytime existence he does it? If you consider the process from a psychological-physiological point of view you will easily notice that a light, partial sleep occurs in the listener. The 'I' and the astral body glide over what they are taking in, they live into it. In listening man steps slightly out of himself. In listening, he slips into a condition that is similar but then again dissimilar to sleep. It is similar to sleep in that the 'I' and astral body are slightly disengaged, dissimilar in that they remain receptive, perceptive and self-aware. Thus the process is extraordinarily similar to imagination. It is a subtle, conscious imagining that is still strongly suppressed in the subconscious. Such is the process at hand.

To every such process there is a reaction within the human being himself; we take this into account as well. Let us look at what takes place in the person who is not reciting. What does he do when he listens? He brings his etheric body into motion. The etheric body reacts. In fact, the etheric body takes up those movements which it carries out—only much more weakly—when the person is asleep and has left his etheric body behind in the physical body. When the human being sleeps the etheric body is considerably more active than when he is awake. During this dampened sleep taking place in the active listener, the movements of the etheric body are awakened to a greater degree. These movements of the etheric body can be observed. In the active listener, we see a person demonstrating in a heightened manner the movements which human beings otherwise carry out in a weakened form during sleep. You can study in the listener, who promptly performs them for you, ether movements of the human being in sleep. It isn't at all necessary to study the person while actually asleep; one can study the etheric movements of the human being when he is actively listening. Here in fact we have the heightened movements of the etheric body in sleep. One studies these movements and has them carried out by the physical body. That is to say, one allows the physical body to glide into all those etheric movements which one has studied in the manner just described. In eurythmy we do what the human being carries out with his etheric body constantly while actively listening. You can see what is actually taking place.

Now that we have observed what actually occurs, its effect will become apparent as well. The result is that through the

detour of the physical movement, you carry over into consciousness what otherwise occurs unconsciously. You
stimulate the astral body and the ego again by means of this
detour through the physical body, and you strengthen them.
But what happens as a result of this? When the astral body
and the 'I' are strengthened in this manner, their activity
becomes similar to the activity in the child and still growing
person as it occurs naturally. You are calling upon the forces
of growth in the human being.[40] You are working directly
into the person's forces of growth. If the person is still a child
and shows signs of being retarded in his growth, you can
stimulate his growth in this way. If the person is no longer a
child, and the forces of growth have already diminished, or if
the person is actually in the second half of life, you call upon
the youthful forces, the rejuvenating forces in him, which
cannot contribute to his growth since the human organism,
of course, is fully developed. We can support a child in his
growth or combat* his abnormal growth by having him do
eurythmy. In the case of the fully grown person, the inner
organism presents too great a resistance to the outer organism for us to be able to make him grow. Nevertheless, we can
still introduce these forces of growth. The result is that,
crashing against the resistance of the organism, they metamorphose; that means, they activate in their metamorphosed
state the sculptural force of the inner organs. They stimulate
the plastic, sculptural force of the inner organs, and these
inner organs learn better to breathe and better to digest.[41]
They are encouraged to stimulate in its entirety the necessary
activity of the human organism.

------

* The German text in the shorthand report *bekämfen*, 'combat', can also be
read as *dämpfen*, 'dampen down'

When artistic eurythmy is carried out one should not think of it in the first instance as eurythmy therapy; nevertheless, in the moment a person begins to be abnormal in any way it will have a therapeutic effect. We have already seen the examples where, when the usual eurythmy is reinforced, the reaction which follows is naturally also strengthened and we can form a mental picture of how this eurythmy affects the sculptural forces of the organization.

You can understand that the habitual practice of eurythmy activates the plasticity of the organs, their sculptural force, and that as a result the human being becomes internally a better breather—in respect to the deeper levels of the inwardly orientated digestion, he becomes a better person, if I may so express myself. He becomes a person who has his whole organism more within his own control. He becomes an inwardly more agile person. And to become a true artist is nothing other than to make the inner man more flexible, supple and agile. That can be seen, for example, when one sculpts. You cannot sculpt properly unless, for example, in experience you transpose yourself into the form that you are developing as a sculpture, unless you bring to life in yourself the forces that are building the form, that express themselves in the form. But when you see the human organism itself as an implement and carry out what corresponds within, then what is the case in outward artistry is in a higher degree the case here as well, for at this point you can do no other than call forth internally what corresponds to the outward movement.

If you would be so good, we will do the poem again now, this time with only the vowels. So that the emphasis is on the vowels alone [*Frl. Wolfram and Frau Dr Steiner*].

What I have just said about the physiology of eurythmy is

specialized here. When only the vowels are carried out, then that which I have characterized does not come to expression in its entirety. What I characterized is correct when someone speaks and the movements are made alternately for the consonants and the vowels. For what we have just done, what I said is not entirely correct—it will have to be specialized. For here specific, differentiated movements have been carried out, all of which prove to be movements within the etheric body, having primarily to do with what lies in the rhythmic system. We fasten our attention on that system which—as an etheric system—participates especially when vowels are spoken.

When a person listens to vowels, which of course occurs in so specialized a manner only in eurythmy, and to which for this reason attention must be drawn, what takes place is especially important therapeutically. One can recite a sequence of vowels for this person, or have him carry out such movements. In the latter case, while doing eurythmy he would be actively listening to the movements which are the expressive forms for the vowel element. In the normal person listening to vowels, those movements of the etheric body corresponding to the rhythmic system become active, in the way already described. So now you have the person doing eurythmy, carrying out in turn those movements through which he glides with his physical body. He glides into those movements, which otherwise take place in the etheric body when vowels are heard. That is how the matter is 'specialized'.

In this way, in particular those organs belonging to the rhythmic system[42] are stimulated, the organs of respiration and the inner activity of digestion. These organs are strengthened; in them the appeal goes out to the forces of growth in the growing child, or alternatively within the organization of the fully grown adult, to the plastic, sculptural forces which are precisely those showing resistance. This will lead you into the physiology of doing vowels in eurythmy. In applying for therapeutic ends everything derived from the vowel element in eurythmy you will be able to affect the rhythmic organs in particular.

Now perhaps Frau Baumann will do the same poem once again consonantally. You will notice at a glance the radical difference between the consonants and the vowels as they are carried out eurythmically. The difference is indeed thoroughly radical. Wishing to study what we have just seen, we will have to make clear to ourselves how the matter would be if in ordinary listening we were to hear only the consonants. For civilized people that is seldom so, but among less civilized peoples it is sometimes the case that they must listen to much of a consonantal nature. The consonantal world in speech is appreciably richer among less civilized peoples, and the transition from one consonant to another is stronger and unilluminated by a vowel lying between. You will find it possible to observe this right into Europe. Just look at words written in the Czech language and you will see just what combinations of consonants are present. To be sure, when the words are spoken the vowel element sounds within these combinations of consonants, but it permeates them only as a continuous, hardly differentiated, undercurrent. And if you listen to Czech you will say to yourself: to listen to this consonantal element is entirely different from listening to a language that is thoroughly permeated by vowels. We have to do with quite another process here, which can be characterized best in the following manner.

As an ordinary listening process, this process strongly calls forth those movements of the etheric body which are otherwise actually carried out in the case of physical movements. They are retained and so, while listening to consonants, the human being lives in a certain tension. Unconsciously, he would like to be imitating outwardly, physically, when he listens to consonants, but he holds back. The situation is alive with tension. A state of pacification prevails, but it is an artificially induced pacification called forth by the power of one's own ego in opposition to those movements which want to be carried out. Volition dammed up* within itself is manifest when consonants are heard. You will consequently find that listening to consonants is inwardly exceptionally invigorating. If one has an eye for it, one can study how peoples such as the Czechs comport themselves inwardly— how the human being deports himself in his interior in relation to these tensions, these aggressive forces, once one knows that they are built up out of the consonantal element of the language. It is a continual curbing of what unceasingly strives to become physical movement.

Once again, it is for the human being a stepping-out, a going-over into the condition of sleep,[43] and this going out, this transition into sleep is extraordinarily interesting. Consider the human being schematically—head, rhythmic system, system of the limbs and the metabolism.

In listening to consonants, the system primarily engaged is the system of the limbs and the metabolism. The person wants to move his limbs, wants to break into movement, but the movement is converted into tension. He passes as it were

---

* In earlier German editions the text read *gestaut*, later revised to *gestaehlt* (steeled).

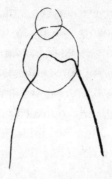

into a state of sleep, which actually does not take place in other respects, for the ego and the astral body—which go out in ordinary sleep—remain within the organism.* One even tries in this case to bring about a kind of artificial sleep for the system of the limbs and the metabolism. But when one falls asleep to a degree in the system of the limbs and the metabolism, a strong reaction makes itself evident. This reaction consists of dreaming. But now, the consciousness is not so organized that one can dream. Dreams, as it were, come into being playing about the human being (orange).

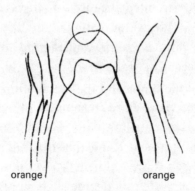

orange   orange

---

* See note 43.

They affect the outer astrality and the outer ether. People who listen to consonants reinforce the aura in their surroundings. This expresses itself in turn in its polarity—what remains here in the subconscious as polar content plays about the head as a factor of volition and feeling, penetrating into the organism of the head (violet).

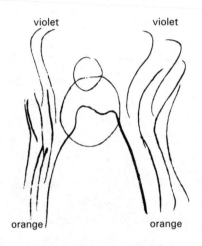

You may notice an intensification of self-assertion and self-will in people who are accustomed to living in the consonantal element. Dreams transformed into will, play through the organism of the head.

What are 'dreams transformed into will' from a physiological point of view? If one examines the etheric-physical correlative, it is essentially what is plastically at work in the organization of the head.[44] The plastic effect on the organization of the head is pre-eminent, and in this manner it will be possible to activate to a degree such an organization of a head, which is as it were retarded. If one has to do with a feeble-minded person, or with someone where it can be demonstrated physically that his head organism is not in order, one should let him do consonants in eurythmy.

One engages oneself with those forces which otherwise work as dream-like will in the entire remaining system of the limbs and the metabolism, which stimulate there the organization and preserve its activity. One makes the heads more active of the feeble-minded and those who are otherwise retarded in their head-organization. So you can employ this kind of eurythmy to arouse therapeutic forces for the organization of the head,[45] particularly when you carry it out in the intensified form, with the strengthened metamorphosis of the consonants,[46] of which we have heard in the last few days. When wishing to consider the physiology of eurythmy, it is natural to keep the active, moving human being in view; we have to pursue a real physiology. In ordinary physiology it is not physiology at all that is actually pursued. Even when an experiment is conducted on the living person, people proceed from the mechanical side; or they start with the corpse and draw conclusions about physiology in actuality. The result is something inferred. If one wishes to attain to a physiology of these processes, what is otherwise inferred has to be read from man's inner activity. It will be seen how this sort of study will quicken the whole of physiology.

Consider alone the following. What is the process of digestion, as observed in the living human being? It is metabolic activity that thrusts itself into the rhythmic activity, which unfolds in the direction of the rhythmic [system]. Digestive activity is metabolic activity which is to a degree caught up by the rhythm of the circulatory organs. A continuing process is taking place here, which is a combination of the metabolic activity in the tissue fluid. When the rhythm pulses up against it,* what is metabolic activity in the tissue fluid passes over into the rhythm of the organs of circulation and is pulled along with it. The more chaotic activity—the chaos astir in the movement of the tissue fluid—is taken over into the rhythm of the circulatory system. Physically, human volition lives where the chaos of the tissue fluid passes over into the regular, rhythmic activity of the circulatory system. One must distinguish this activity of will, which consists in the continual transition taking place between the chaotic vigour in the tissue fluid and the rhythmically regular, harmonizing activity present in the circulatory being, distinguish this from the outer activity into which it pours. It is in this way, nevertheless, that the inner world of man lying within the skin brings itself into harmony with his outer being. Through the subordination of his own being† man incorporates himself into the being of the outer world.[47] Consequently, when you influence this activity through eurythmy—as we have seen with the consonants—you in fact counter the human being's tendency to become self-willed, to become egoistic, and his tendency to become organically egoistic as well. What does it actually mean when man becomes egoistic? Organically expressed it means that the force of plasticity in the organs is diminished and the rigidifying, crystallizing tendency takes the upper hand. The organs no longer want to be modellers,[48] they want to become more crystalline. This tendency can be counteracted by means of consonantal eurythmy.

---

* The German text has *heranschlägt*, 'beating on'; the shorthand could be read as *heraufschlägt*, 'beating upwards'.

† *Eigenwesen*, 'own being' according to the shorthand report, taken in earlier editions as *Innenwesen*, 'inner being'.

Here you have an insight deep into the human organism. Egoists are always people whose stomach, liver and lobes of the lungs threaten to take on a proper wedge-form. They want to become wedges, to become crystalline, whereas in the case of people who are pathologically selfless these organs effuse. They have no crystallizing agency; possessing plastic forces they become round. That is also a pathological condition. It is always the swing of the pendulum from one extreme to the other to which we have to pay heed.

Consider what spiritual activity is. When man thinks and, from out of his thinking, feels—that is designated as spiritual activity in normal life. It is carried out by the most physical part of the head-organism and, for precisely this reason, it is the sublimating spiritual activity, on the one side the individualizing [activity] and on the other side the abstractly felt. When the human being carries out this activity, what happens then? He draws out of his organism the force that enables him to incorporate himself into the outer world. He draws out of his organism the force that, pathologically, entices him to effuse. He makes a crystallizer of himself when he is spiritually active. Certain peoples, the more northern peoples in particular, have developed a strong instinctive consciousness for these matters. In accordance with this instinctive consciousness, they have to date [1921] shown no inclination to introduce eurythmy. Instead, they employ what is more outwardly physiological—Swedish gymnastics, and so on.[49] Nevertheless, they make decided use of the characteristic alternating effect, by alternating the activity which the children must carry out in scientific study in school—when they must think and so on—with what diverts them to movement. They expect every teacher to be a gymnastic teacher as well, and require on the other hand that the gymnastic instructor stands at the spiritual level of the child. Such things should be taken into consideration in an advanced civilization. However, if I may make a statement that may appear to be a bit sharp—though it is meant only to enlighten—one must take time if one wishes to take these matters into account instinctively. Such things must be carried out by those peoples who take less part in the process of civilization, who live a life apart, more for themselves, and who are thus able gradually to develop instinctively that which has to do with the rhythm of spiritual and physical activity. The Swedes and the Norwegians who lead a more isolated existence, for example, can put such ideas instinctively into practice particularly well. For others the practice of such matters must be more conscious, since these peoples are more engaged in the general world processes—people, for example, who must concern themselves (as was of late very much the case) with making war, and so on. These peoples must see these matters much more consciously. And those who stand in the centre of the world's movement, who have to take part in its affairs while the world, so to speak, turns around them, they will soon see what they will leave behind if they do not turn to these things consciously. They will gradually degenerate. That is something that Switzerland in particular should take to heart.

These things can be observed to play a part in the state of the world as a whole. The general conditions prevailing in the world, my dear friends, are of course the result of human activity, yet even today they proceed more from unconscious human activity than from conscious activity. We are given the task, however, gradually to transmute man's unconscious activity into conscious activity.

How does this spiritual activity work in man? It awakens

the crystallizing forces. In people with weak egos it strengthens the 'I', it makes the ego more egoistic. In people who effuse organically because they are not sufficiently egoistic, we will find it necessary to activate the forces of egoism—not for the benefit of the soul, but for the organism. We could stimulate these forces by outward means as well. It would be natural to advise people who effuse organically to consume substances containing sugar. However, they sometimes have an antipathy here—a fact which expresses the true state of affairs.

However, that is something of much less interest to us at the moment. What interests us just now is that through the vowel element in eurythmy we have the possibility of working most effectively in this direction. You can bring the human being organically to himself through doing vowels in eurythmy. You can awaken the forces that bring him to himself organically. For certain people this will be most necessary, among them sleepy-headed people. You will find that the alternation between the two, between the vowels and the consonants in eurythmy, will work favourably as well, as it induces a living rhythm in the human being such as should exist between opening oneself to the world and retracting into oneself. That will be called forth by alternating consonantal elements and vowel elements in eurythmy.

It is particularly important, of course, when you intend to apply eurythmy for therapeutic purposes, to make your own what I would like to call this physiological-psychological perception of what actually takes place. You should understand that the person who does consonantal eurythmy tends to call forth around himself a sort of aura that works back on him, bringing him out of a vacant merging with the world. In the case of the person who does vowels in eurythmy, his aura is drawn together, densified in itself, which is of course always the case with spiritual activity as well, and that the inner organs are thus stimulated to bring the person to himself.

Educationally considered, through alternating between the lessons, one would place in the morning hours subjects where more mental work would be done. The lessons in which there would be more movement and where a great deal of eurythmy would be done call forth rhythmic activity in the growing child that has an extraordinarily beneficial effect. All the detriments that are of necessity incurred through an overly strong mental exertion are balanced out by doing eurythmy. For this reason eurythmy has an especially bene-ficial function within the curriculum as a whole.[50]

What I have to say particularly to the physicians about eurythmy I will include in the course of my lectures to them. So we conclude our consideration of eurythmy as such here. Tomorrow there will be two consecutive medical lectures, where the eurythmists will not be present.

[*At the conclusion of this series of lectures, a vote of thanks was expressed by Dr Friedrich Husemann.[51] Because of the references to eurythmy therapy in the second lecture held on the following day, 18 April 1921, it was included in GA 315 and the earlier English translation as 'Lecture 7', which follows below. 'Lecture 8' was held the following year in Stuttgart.*]

We stand today at the end of this lecture course and it cer-tainly is everybody's wish once more to look back on it. I believe we have all felt that, especially with this course of lectures, a certain climax was given of what we have received so far from Herr Dr Steiner as stimuli for medicine. That it was possible to hold a lecture course for physicians and artists seems to be a symbol as it were of that which we actually want in our anthroposophical striving in medicine. That this synthesis could come about is perhaps a fulfilment, too, of what Goethe says pictorially in his *Wilhelm Meister*, that one should not let the medical students carry out so much anatomy but rather to synthesize. One should teach them to put together again the human body out of the individual muscles, bones and organs, and out of this feeling of reassembling the sound feeling of healing would arise.

This, I believe, has been placed before us with this lecture course, how the possibility of the synthetic, integrated thinking and feeling can be stimulated in us and that precisely such a lecture course, which shows how the word, how the spiritual element, goes over into movement, into the body, should stimulate us into action and not to mere talking. This actually lies in the whole tendency in what has been given to us here.

In this there now lies a small difficulty, since especially where one feels stimulated into action one can start doing too much. It can happen that all the stimuli which have been given here will be used a lot, all over the place. Here our [Medical] Association has specially asked that we take seriously what Herr Dr Steiner has repeatedly emphasized, that we look at these therapeutic indications as therapeutic means. That means that they should be used under the guidance and collaboration of a medical doctor, not blindly used, because that could lead to serious mishaps. On the other hand, we have to think that everything that appears dilettante will come out in public, severely damaging us and our Movement.

Consequently, I would like you to take really seriously the

admonishments that Herr Dr Steiner has put to you in this regard. What has been given here has to be digested by us, but this can only happen in a fruitful way when we work together, just as we have been together here. So I would like to conclude by conveying our thanks to Herr Dr Steiner, especially expressing that we really will work further on these things, not only taking up work in our Movement, but precisely with understanding.

Lecture 7

Dornach, 18 April 1921 (held before physicians)

What I have to say in relation to eurythmy, my respected friends, with regard to particulars, you will find it necessary to elucidate what I have to tell you today about eurythmy through your knowledge of physiology, and so on. How that can be done will reveal itself as if of its own accord, if I may say so. When we look into a spiritual-corporeal process such as that which takes place in eurythmy, we can do no other than indicate the deeper spiritual-physical context. So I would like to draw your attention to the following.

First, we must contemplate the extra-human world-process, which one usually traces only in its details and not in regard to what is actually inwardly active. Just consider what earth-formation is, in reality: a formative tendency works inward from the planetary sphere. Furthermore, a formative working into the earth takes place from what lies beyond the planetary sphere—continuous, radiant cosmic forces expressing themselves in powerful entities, radiating towards the earth.

In this context, we may conceive of these cosmic powers as working towards the centre, building up from without that which is on and in the earth—although they could encompass as well all that I have said earlier about such raying. We could conceive them like this. The fact is that, for example, the whole metallic part of the earth, the entire metals[52] are not in essence formed out of some force or other within the earth, but are actually set into the earth out of the cosmos. Now,

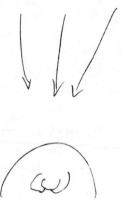

these forces that work through the ether can be called formative forces, formative forces working in from outside. They
do not work from the planets—for in that case they would
work from a centre. The planets are there, that is, the
planetary sphere, for the specific purpose of modifying these
forces. Please take note of them in precisely this context of the
formative forces. In opposition to them stand those forces in
the human being and in the earth which take up those formative forces, consolidating them. They assemble them
around a point so that the earth can come into being. We may
call those forces which consolidate, the consolidating forces.*

In the human being they are present as the forces that
plastically build up the organs, whereas the other forces, the
formative forces, have more to do with propelling the organs
out of the spiritual-etheric world into the physical world.
That is a process which becomes so tangible in the contrast
between the propulsive powers of magnesium and the
rounding-off forces of fluorine.[53] It is a process active

---

* *Kräfte des Befestigens*—the *consolidating* forces could also be translated as
binding or *anchoring* forces.

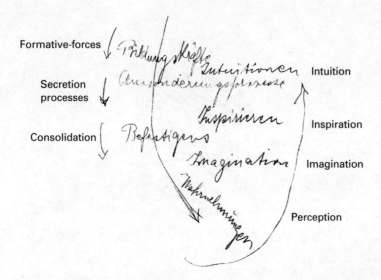

everywhere, in the teeth from below upwards and rounding-off at the top, but from front to back as well and from the back forwards, from above to below, rounding-off down below. This process will become directly tangible (as I'd like to say again), if you picture to yourself that, in association with the tendency to push something spherical forwards, from without inwards, something is formed which is opposed by a process of spherical formation from below upwards [in the following sketch].

Between these two processes is that which mediates: on the one hand processes of secretion, and on the other hand the absorption of other (*von andern*) [secretions], and so on—which can be called processes of secretion in the widest sense. In the final analysis, absorption is dependent upon a secretion inwards, which is in turn re-absorbed. In between lies what can best be called excretory processes.

Such an excretory process becomes once again tangible

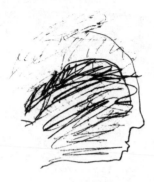

when you picture to yourself on the one side what continually wants to excrete carbon [orange in the sketch] and what takes it up through respiration from the front (*von vorne*) in the formation of carbon dioxide [white].

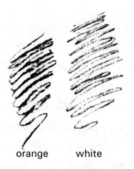

orange   white

Behind* this such a process of excretion is continuing. When you descend further into the system of the metabolism and the limbs, you have a proper process of consolidating. However, this process is present in the other direction as well. You will be able to follow it most tangibly by studying

---

* In the stenograph the word could be read as *dahinter*, 'behind' or *dahinunter*, 'below'.

the eye, which is built inwards from without, as embryology demonstrates, but is consolidated from within. The formation is internalized. That is the manner in which the eye develops. It is internalized.

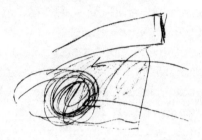

As we progress to that which is of soul and spirit in man, to the organs of the soul and spirit, to the sense-organs, we find that the process of consolidation has become spiritualized, truly ensouled and spiritualized in perception. That is, more or less, the descending process which leads to the formation of the organs [see sketch on page 91]. We find at the lowermost end the process of sensory perception, perception of objects. If this development continues, goes further in this direction, then the process of perception encounters the consolidating forces. Should it become conscious in this encounter, it will become Imagination. If Imagination develops further and becomes conscious in encountering the process of secretion, it becomes Inspiration. And when Inspiration develops further in the direction of the formative forces, collides with them consciously and so comprehends them, it becomes Intuition. One can develop this progression in the life of the soul stage by stage from perception of sensory objects to Imagination, to Inspiration and to Intuition.

Intuition: Formative-forces
Inspiration: Secretion processes
Imagination: Consolidation
Perception

This process unfolding in the soul, however, is based on the process of coming-into-being. As you can see here, it is but the inverse of this process of becoming. You encounter what has become, rising into this becoming in the opposite direction. Formation takes place in the descending direction. The human being ascends in the opposite direction; he advances to meet what is coming into being. What one develops as powers of perception and cognition in Imagination, Inspiration and Intuition always has its counter-activity in the creative powers, in the creative powers which express themselves in the formative forces, in the processes of secretion and of consolidation. From all of this you will gather that what is active in the human organism in the opposite direction, in its coming-into-being, is that into which one ascends when rising in knowledge. You will perceive that in reality what we attain in Imagination are the same powers which, without our being conscious of them, reveal themselves in the phenomena of growth, in the plastic phenomena of growth. If we ascend to Inspiration, we come upon the forces which inspire man from without inwards in his breathing, which shape him through and through as he breathes, which shape themselves into the plastic forces as they work through these forces, to a degree. And if we ascend to Intuition, we rise in reality to the Primal Mover (*Agens*) who enters into our plastic forms from the world without as substantial Being.

You see, in this way we grasp the human being as he takes

shape out of the cosmos.[54] If we apply the knowledge we have gained in one way or another through anatomy or physiology and illuminate it with what is given us here, then we begin to understand the organs and their functions. This is an indication of how to understand the organs and their functions. So, in that which is always at work plastically on the human being, what normally permeates plastically through and through the human being—here yesterday's lecture will be a help—lives on the other hand in the movements for the consonants, the unconscious imaginative forces which call forth a streaming*[55] through of the organism (as I said yesterday). Here you can perceive how consonantal eurythmy takes hold of deficient formative powers, deficient plastic forces in the human being, transforming them into something truly sculptural.

Let us assume we have a child and we see that the plasticity is deficient, that plasticity [*die Plastik*] is proliferating too strongly. What does it mean, when we say that plasticity is growing without control? It means that the plasticity is working centrifugally, thus making the head large, because it is working centrifugally, and in doing so is no longer permitting the head to be permeated in the proper manner with imaginative forces. These must be supplied. So one will let the child do consonantal eurythmy.

Question: 'A two-year-old boy has a large head, is nevertheless not hydrocephalic and is otherwise apparently healthy.'
Here you have the effective antidote, in properly applied consonantal eurythmy. Here we have arrived at the point at which a thorough observation of the morphology, of the more

---

* The shorthand can be read as *Durchströmen*, 'streaming through', or *Durchträumen*, 'dreaming through'.

profound morphological facts, can provide a direct indication for the eurythmical treatment.

Another question: 'A boy, twelve and three-quarters years of age, whose growth in height is distinctly retarded, with no organic findings other than worms; intelligent but intellectually quickly tired.'
A most interesting complex of symptoms, all of which indicate that the imaginative forces are insufficient, that the plastic forces in the organs are proliferating because of a lack of inner plastic forces, of plastic soul-forces. These plastic forces of the soul are those which destroy parasites. It is no wonder that when these forces are insufficient the child has worms. [Gap in stenograph] Thus one should have him do consonantal eurythmy; therein lies the antidote. These associations will provide you with concrete indications of where you can employ eurythmy. Although the phenomena are somewhat camouflaged here, eurythmy will have an extraordinarily positive effect even in such cases, particularly if one complements it medicinally.

Here I have an interesting question that has been presented to me. Naturally I must answer the questions in principle. If complications of any sort should appear, they can later be taken into special consideration as the case demands. However, although it may be necessary to combine something else along with it, the matter has nevertheless been thoroughly dealt with from the side characterized.

'I have as a patient, a five-year-old child who lost a great deal of blood as the result of a bullet wound suffered in the outbreaks of violence; two years ago a deformation of the joints set in . . . [Gap in stenograph] (These are things which could lead to anaemia

and similar conditions in adults.) How could one help this child therapeutically?'

Here you have a deformation of the joints. That is an outwardly working tendency of plastic forces that are unable to remain within. So these forces ray outwards, leaving the human being instead of working within him as they should. They will be reflected in the most effective manner precisely through the practice of consonantal eurythmy. In doing consonantal eurythmy you will call forth the objectively effective imaginations that offset the deformations. As the manner in which the question is placed quite correctly indicates, people in the future will in general tend to be deformed in the most manifold ways, because they will no longer be able to build up the normalizing human form out of* the involuntarily active forces. Man will become free; he will gradually become free even in respect to the building up of his own form. However, he must then be able to do something with this freedom. He must go on to engender imaginations that continuously counter the deformation.

Now as to the other case, you see that we are here concerned with a dearth of objective Imagination. We could have to do with a deficiency of objective Inspiration as well, which would express itself in a deformation of the rhythmic system, if I may call it that. In the case of a deformation of the rhythmic system, the objective Inspiration which goes inwards does not encounter the circulatory rhythm in the proper manner. One can work towards normalizing the situation by practising vowels in eurythmy. In eurythmy the vowels affect internal irregularities which are precisely not accompanied by morphological changes, even as con-

---

* In the stenograph can be read as *auf* or *in*.

sonantal eurythmy affects deformations and the tendency to deformation.

As I said earlier, it may nevertheless be necessary to render aid when something appears in particularly radical form, as in the case of the deformations of the joints that we just discussed. There it would be necessary to come to the assistance of the consonantal eurythmical process thera-peutically. This consonantal process works by stimulating through its Imagination the inner breathing of the organs orientated from without inwards and lying on the far side of the intestinal wall—the lungs, the kidneys, the liver, and so on. When a person does consonantal eurythmy, it is a fact that particularly the back of the head, the lungs, the liver and the kidneys begin to sparkle and flash; something is really there that indicates the reaction of the spirit and soul to what is done outside in the consonants. The whole human being becomes a shining being in these organs, and the movements that are carried out are in continuous opposition to the luminous movements within, and in particular there appears (I would like to say) an entire luminous reproduction of the secretory process of the kidneys through certain consonantal movements. One has a picture of the secretory process of the kidneys in this luminous process which comes about as the result of consonantal eurythmy. That works over into the unconscious imaginations. And the whole process in which this part begins to shine is the same process that I described as being especially under the influence of copper. It is the same process. Here one must draw the attention of the physicians to the fact that there are people with particular forms of illness. These forms of illness were again brought to my attention yesterday when I was shown some painted pictures, very much admired in some quarters at least, and was asked whether they were particularly 'occult'. In a certain sense, of course, they are occult, but it is extraordinarily difficult to speak to people about these things, for they are an objectively fixed kidney efflorescence; they are the objectively fixed process of the excretion of urine. When in the case of persons predisposed to this illness the process of urinary excretion becomes an abnormal, luminous process, that is, when the process of excretion halts—a purely metabolic ill-ness—the kidneys then begin to shine. When this inwardly directed clairvoyance then sets in, people begin to draw wildly. What they produce will be aesthetic, in an outer formal manner beautiful in every case. The colours applied will be beautiful. But, of course, people are not content when one says to them, 'Yes, there you have painted something very beautiful; it is in fact your congested urinary secretion.' I can assure you that congested urinary secretion and sup-pressed sexual desires—which lead as well, in a certain way, to metabolic irregularities—are often presented by people of particularly mystical nature, as mystically profound drawings and paintings. In much of what makes its appearance in the world in this manner one should recognize the symptoms of pathological abnormalities in the human being that are still just bearable.

As you see, anthroposophically orientated spiritual science is not mysticism as mysticism is commonly under-stood, since it fosters no illusions about matters such as we have just characterized. Quite the contrary, it investigates just such matters. People, however, take exception to one for doing this. They resent my having gone so far in a public lecture as to indicate that the lovely poetry, for example, of Mechthild von Magdeburg[56] and of St Theresa,[57] are the inspirational reflexes of processes arising from repressed sexuality. Here, of course, the things are not drawn or painted, but poetically expressed. Naturally it is not pleasant for people to hear Mechthild von Magdeburg or St Theresa described as personalities with a strong sexuality, which they restrained precisely because it was too strong for them, that certain metabolic-circulatory processes resulted from this retention, and that the reactions to this in turn appeared in such a form that they were fixed in very beautiful poetry. Indeed, this phenomenon leads extraordinarily deep into the mysteries of existence, when considered in a higher light. However, one must be able to rise to such an interpretation. Consequently, one must have at least a notion of these peculiar processes which light up as inward processes when eurythmy is done outwardly. And in the moment when what is concealed within the poetry becomes eurythmy, as I showed you yesterday—when a beautiful poem is read and the eurythmy corresponding to it is done as we saw yesterday in vowels or consonants—then the one thing crosses the other. An inward, silent speaking joins what is carried out outwardly in movements, in the person doing eurythmy as well. When this process does not exude in sultry poetry but takes instead the course of accompanying beautiful poetry as eurythmy, then that which takes place in the human being does not become a recording of mysticism, but a definite process of healing for the human being. One can say that when one lets the patients do eurythmy in such a manner that one continually brings to his attention, 'Listen carefully, bring intensely into consciousness the sound that you hear, the relationships of the sentence you hear, to which you are doing eurythmy', then one will initiate his ascent to the outward formative forces, to the objectively intuiting powers. When one wants to

affect all that has remained in the human being from what
no longer took place between birth and death, but what
materialism calls 'heredity'[58]—the greater part of which,
however, is carried over from the pre-existent spiritual soul-
life—if one wants to affect what can be called congenital
defects, and so on, then one will do well to work (particularly during the course of youth) repeatedly through
eurythmy by challenging the person doing it: 'Make very
clear to yourself what you hear outwardly!' By this method
one can drive out all the tendencies to fix inwardly what
would like to arise and take form in something like mystical
poetry or mystical drawing. Precisely that will be connected
to the beautiful outer poem. It is the reverse process. A true
mystic knows that what of an abnormal nature is reflected
by the human being as beauty always has a questionable
side. By contrast, one cannot claim that when what is
beautiful in the outer world is experienced inwardly it
appears as a particularly magnificent and beautiful picture.
On the contrary, it becomes schematic and thereby
abstract—abstract as if it were sketched, abstract as a drawing is abstract. That is precisely what is healthy, however,
and what is desired. The beautiful historic process would
not have taken place, but if, for example, Mechthild von
Magdeburg had been instigated to do eurythmy to good
poetry, her entire mystic fate would have been spared her.
Naturally one can say here that a point has been reached
where in a certain sense good and evil cease to exist; one
enters into the amoral sphere of Nietzsche's *Beyond Good
and Evil*.[59] Of course, one cannot be so philistine as to claim
that all the Mechthilds von Magdeburg should be eradi-
cated, roots and branch! On the other hand, when people
attempt to prevent this tendency from undue proliferation,

you may be certain that from the supersensory worlds care will be taken that the corresponding connections with these supersensory worlds nevertheless remain.

Although it is quite late, I would still like to go into a few matters in order perhaps to bring some clarification. I would like to start with the following question:

'Couldn't the therapeutic eurythmy exercises be reinforced by rational breathing exercises? It needn't necessarily be hatha yoga.'[60]

To this I would like to make the following remarks. In our times, and within the direction that the continually progressing human nature has taken, rational breathing exercises, as a reinforcement of the eurythmical exercises, can in fact only be treated in the following manner. It will be observed that a tendency towards a modification in the rhythm of respiration arises of its own accord under the influence of the vowels in eurythmy. One will notice this quite clearly. Here we find ourselves in the uncomfortable situation that we should avoid stereotyping, avoid saying the one thing or another in general, but should first observe what is to be done. Concern yourself in each individual case with the breathing of the person in whose healing you are attempting to be of assistance by means of eurythmical vowel exercises. Observe the modification of the breathing and subsequently make the patient aware that he can consciously pursue this tendency himself. We are no longer human beings like the ancient orientals, who would go the reverse route and influence the entire human being by way of a prescribed method of breathing. This is something which today leads of necessity, in every case, to inner shocks, no matter how it is prescribed; it should really be avoided. We just have to learn to notice what kind of effect eurythmy itself, especially the vowels in eurythmy, has on the breathing process. And then we can consciously continue the tendency that arises eurythmically in the individual case. You will certainly observe that this respiratory process will be carried on individually, continued in varying manners in different people.

My esteemed friends, those are more or less the things that it is possible to answer at the moment. We have no real possibility of dealing with a number of matters that have got bogged down due to the shortness of time. In closing, my dear friends, I want to warn you that you must be prepared that your medical colleagues in the world will wage their wars no less intensely when they become aware of your bringing something of our sort to bear. You will need the penetrating power of conviction to weaken what will confront you. In no case, of course, may what you are confronted with lead you to neglect these matters; we may permit ourselves no illusions about those antagonistic forces we arouse.

At the end of this lecture course, I would as well like to state that in order to make the movement possible—as it should now be inaugurated in the medical field—I will adhere everywhere to the policy of not involving myself directly with the patients in the therapeutic process, but will discuss and consult only with the physicians themselves. You will always be in the position to refute any allegations that I myself interfere in any way in an unjustified manner in the therapy. I have already mentioned this at the end of the previous lecture course. This has been made extraordinarily difficult for me even from the anthroposophical side—this cannot be passed over in silence—as people naturally make all possible demands in this direction. It is also definitely the case that among anthroposophists the tendency exists not only *not* to rise above egoism, but sometimes to become even more egoistic than normal people are. Then when the occasion arises it is often a matter of complete indifference to the person what the welfare of the movement may entail. That is, the welfare of the movement is dependent in each individual instance upon a rejection of the practice of what the world outside terms quackery, that a healing process should take place in the whole of medicine and should not be disturbed by the demands arising from an individual's personal aspirations. People will make it difficult, but it must be carried through in this direction since we will only be able to succeed in this area when we can stand up to the outer world—as we are otherwise able to, in the anthroposophical movement, in so far as matters are conducted with understanding and not bowdlerized by people without understanding. Simply by virtue of knowing what is going on in the anthroposophical movement we must be in the position to say, 'What is being said there [in the outer world] is certainly a lie, it is beyond doubt an invention.' We must simply always be in the position to say that, in certain cases. We come to be able to say that, when we are all inwardly initiated into the contents of matters such as those to which I have drawn attention here, that I myself do not intervene in the therapeutic process, but that within the anthroposophical movement the doctors are responsible for the therapy of the patients.

Having said what was necessary, I want to add nothing more than the wish that the stimuli—which, in this lecture course in particular, have often remained mere indications—

may work on in you and become active in the appropriate manner for the welfare of humanity. Hopefully we will have the opportunity to carry on in some manner what we have already twice begun; in any case we will make an effort to carry on with it. With this wish, my dear friends, I will close these contemplations, in the hope that our deeds in these directions may be in accord with our wishes. It was very satisfying to see you here. It will be a satisfying feeling to think back on these days here, which it was your desire to spend together towards the enrichment of medical science. The thoughts that hold us together will accompany you, my dear friends, on the paths that you will tread, to transform into deeds what we attempted to activate, initially here, as thoughts.

Words of appreciation were expressed at the end of the lecture course by Prof. Dr med. et Dr. med. dent. Oskar Römer.[61]

Lecture 8

(held during the 'Medical Week', Stuttgart,
28 October 1922)

The wish has been expressed for me to expound somewhat further upon eurythmy therapy. Basically, the empirical material relating to eurythmy therapy was developed and presented in the recent lecture course for physicians in Dornach,[62] and it is hardly necessary to go beyond what was given at that time. Used in the proper manner, it will be of far-reaching importance. Today, I would like to speak to you about the whole purpose and meaning of eurythmy therapy.

Eurythmy therapy took shape, in a certain way, out of something purely artistic, out of what was first developed as an artistic impulse. In certain contexts a basis for the correct understanding of eurythmy therapy has to be taken from artistic eurythmy. Now perhaps I will be most clearly understood if I attempt initially to indicate the difference between artistic eurythmy and eurythmy therapy. Eurythmy in general is based on the possibility of transforming in a certain direction what takes place in the human organism in speech. For this reason, eurythmy is in the first place artistically really a kind of visible speech. We recognize two components working together in human speech. One component originates through a particular use of the formative apparatus (of which I may speak on the basis of the preceding lectures), from a layer of the nervous system which lies further inward. What is related to the mental image plays in here.

Essentially, the apparatus of mental representation in the speech apparatus extends, to be sure in a somewhat complicated way, even into the construction of the nervous system. It is precisely this which then produces in its further radiation one of the components at work in speech. The other component arises out of the human being's metabolism. In a way, we have a meeting of two dynamic systems, the one coming out of the human metabolism and the other arising from the nerve-sensory system. The two encounter each other in such a way that the metabolic system is transformed first into the circulatory processes; that which has to do with mental representation, coming from the nerve-sensory system, is metamorphosed into the respiratory system. In the respiratory and circulatory systems these two dynamic systems converge and, since the whole is carried over into the air by means of the speech-system, it is possible for the human astral organism to stream into what is created there as movement of the air. If we consider the outermost periphery of the human organism, we see that speech comes into being through an embodiment on the one hand of what has to do with mental picturing and, on the other, of the metabolic nature. This latter, when expressed in terms of the soul, is actually of will-nature—what is expressed in the soul as will and is expressed bodily in the metabolic system, that is, to the extent that the nervous system has a part in the will. This in fact it has, in so far as metabolism takes place—not as nerve-sensory activity—in the nervous system. So there conjoins what is of a volitional nature and finds its bodily expression in the metabolic system, and what is of the nature of mental representation finding its expression in what I would like to call a section or stratum of the nerve-sensory system. They conjoin to form what results. This finds physical expression in what manifests as ordinary speech and singing. In the case of singing it is something different but nonetheless similar. In eurythmy you block out what is of the nature of mental representation to the greatest possible degree and bring volition into force. In this way ordinary speech is metamorphosed into movements of the entire human organism. You strengthen one component, the will or the metabolism, you weaken the mental representation or the nerve-sensory side, and the result is eurythmy. In this way one is really in the position to create correlatives in human movement for the individual sounds, whether they be vowels or consonants. Just as a certain formation and movement of the air can correspond to an 'A' or an 'L', so can an outwardly visible form in movement correspond to an 'A' or an 'L'. Here we have a movement, or movement-structure (as I would like to call it), derived from the human organism through sensory-supersensory vision. This proceeds from the human organism with the same lawfulness as speech in sounds; although more volitionally oriented, it is but a metamorphosis of this speech. One can compose the entire alphabet in this speech; one can bring everything linguistic to expression through this eurythmy. When artistic eurythmy is presented, the attention of the human being and all the processes in the human physical, etheric and astral organisms, which mediate this alertness, are directed to the corresponding sound, to the formation of the word or the artistic formation of the sentence, to the metric form, the poetic form, and so on. When active in artistic eurythmy, you are completely absorbed in the possibilities of artistic formation and portrayal of the elements of speech. The human being surrenders to the outer world when he is artistically active in eurythmy, since in eurythmy you naturally follow the structure that is also common to speech. Since one does not stop at an 'A' or an 'L' in the middle of a word, but carries on further, in artistic eurythmy we have something that may quite possibly take place in the normally functioning human organism. Normal artistic eurythmy has no other physiological consequences for the human organism other than the fact that this artistic eurythmy in an energetic manner calls forth an inner harmony in the human functions, in so far as these functions form a totality in the human organism.

We can say that when we refrain in the right manner from exaggeration in eurythmical artistic activity, it is conducive to health. But just as everything conducive to health can also make one sick if exaggerated, the artistic practice of eurythmy can be overdone. Professor Benedikt,[63] the famous criminal psychologist, because he could not bear the anti-alcohol movement, repeatedly emphasized that more people die from water than from alcohol. Even the statistics must concede that over-indulgence in water leads to numerous sorts of illness. Eurythmy, in general, as long as it remains within the appropriate limits, can only be conducive to health; a certain artistic feeling of satisfaction or dissatisfaction will arise in any case.

That which lives in the devotion to the formations of sound, word and sentence in artistic eurythmy is reflected inwards in eurythmy therapy. It is reflected inwards simply through the fact that in eurythmy therapy the sound 'A', for example, must be repeated a number of times in succession. By this means, something entirely different is achieved than when I pass over from the sound 'A' to an 'I', or something else in an artistic presentation. Now it will be a question of gaining insight into the actual therapeutic process which can take place through eurythmy. I cannot avoid expressing

concern about something which lies close at hand here—
amateurs and dilettantes appropriate such things very easily.
From the beginning I have emphasized that eurythmy therapy should be practised by the doctor him/herself, or at the
very least should only be practised in the most intimate
collaboration with a doctor. The attitude which spiritual
science takes in relation to such offshoots will be taken as
indicative of the position of spiritual science in regard to
medicine as a whole.

Spiritual science does not operate in the field of medicine
in such a manner as I once encountered 20 years ago. People
who called themselves nature-therapy doctors were present
at an anthroposophical convention and presented me with a
treatise in which it was repeatedly stated in a variety of ways
that all healing is based upon bringing into harmony what is
inharmonious in the organism. This sentence was repeated
for six pages in the most manifold variations—one should
'harmonize the disharmonious'. There is nothing at all that
one can object to in this sentence, it is only that one must be
able to do it in a specific manner in a particular case. That is
where it becomes unpleasant for people who hold an opinion
such as was expressed in their final sentence, that everything
that has been said above proves that one can leave the
unbelievably complicated medicine behind and restrict
oneself to harmonizing the disharmonious. That would be, in
their own words, 'intoxicatingly simple'. Something so
intoxicatingly simple I cannot offer you! Medicine cannot be
driven into intoxicating simplicity by spiritual science, but
rather to greater complexity, as you will have gathered by
now from various instances. Through spiritual science you
will not have less to learn, but more, but there is a snag
attached to learning less anyway, because through learning

more everything will become clearer and more ordered, and the learning thereby becomes more interesting. Whoever had the idea that healing would be made easier through spiritual science will already have been convinced by the expositions I have made here that this is not the case.

And so it is with eurythmy therapy. It is definitely the case that eurythmy therapy should not be applied without a thorough diagnosis. It should only be practised in agreement with professional medical science, for the reason that one is dealing here with the application of an exceedingly intimate knowledge of the human organism. Because of the fact that in normal speech the metabolic activity and the plastic activity of the nerve-sensory system collide with one another, the result of this collision is unloaded to the movement of the air—this is something which takes place in relative isolation from the human organism so that as a result speech is released from the organism—all of what is shaped through eurythmy therapy is thrown back into the organism. So we have to do with the following. Imagine that you place an 'A'-movement together with an 'L'-movement. First of all you have the movements repeated, so that the whole affair is not discharged outside, but rather that the repetition pours into the inner processes of the human organism. By allowing the vowel element and consonantal element to work together, let us say in the 'A'-movement and the 'L'-movement, you will always induce a functioning in the human organism that implies a mutual activity of the metabolic man and the nerve-sensory man. To be sure, the activity of the nerve-sensory system is in any case weakened in eurythmy, but the two components, the dampened nerve-sensory activity and the heightened metabolic activity brought about by the eurythmical movement, nevertheless work together in this exceptional proportion. When one does the 'L'-movement repeatedly, and when the 'L'-movement is associated with an 'A'-form, one has simply a driving of the metabolic man against the nerve-sensory-man. Thus one can say: the instigation of the necessary forms and movements carries along the entire functioning of the human organism. When, for example, you let someone carry out a consonantal movement, it works initially by essentially unloading its whole strength, its inner dynamic, onto the process of inhalation; then you actually have the whole process of inhalation in your control. According to the consonants you induce, you have the entire process of in-breathing in your hands. You strengthen the process of inhalation through each consonantal activity.

You perhaps know from what has already been related about eurythmy therapy that movements of artistic eurythmy are somewhat modified for eurythmy therapy. One can say that when an 'A'-movement or an 'L'-movement is carried out, it is always associated with a strengthening or weakening of the thrust initiated by inhalation. Here you have to take inhalation into consideration in its entirety. In examining the in-breathing, we must initially follow its path into the middle part of the human organism, and then through the medial canal, the vertebral canal, into the brain. The activity of the brain is in essence the harmonizing of the breathing activity, in its refinement within the brain, with the nerve-sensory activity. There is no activity of the brain that may be considered alone; every such activity results from the nerve-sensory activity and the breathing activity. All the activities of the brain must be studied in such a way that respiration is taken into consideration. By inducing certain consonants, various consonants, you can, via the breathing, influence the human sculptural, sculpting activity, in the most striking manner.

In the case of a child who is getting his second teeth,[64] for example, you have only to know from a certain artistic grasp of the human organism how the upper teeth will be built up out of sculptural activity which works from above downwards. In the case of the upper teeth, the sculptural activity that forms them is active from the front backwards. How will the lower teeth be formed? In the teeth of the lower jaw the sculptural activity works from the back to the front. If I were to express schematically the activity going on in teething, it would be as follows. The upper teeth are built up from front to back; the back surfaces are shaped and the front surfaces are deposited. The lower teeth are built up from back to front. This is the manner in which the forces work together.

If you notice that a child is experiencing difficulties in teething, you can assist the process in the maxilla, for example, simply by having the child do the movement for 'A'. You can support the same process in the lower jaw with the 'O'-movement. You can in fact get your hands on the sculpting forces through specific effects. In order to give this sculpting activity nourishment, so to speak, you must direct your attention principally to supporting the thrust that accompanies the inhalation; you must add to the sculpting activity accomplished in this way by the 'A'- and 'O'-movements what you observe resulting from the entire human constitution. Let us say we have a person with weak peristalsis, who is somewhat inclined to constipation. In the period of life in which teething takes place, the intestinal activity is related to the building up of the teeth. We focus our attention there, where irregularities in teething have their origin. If you wish to come to the assistance of the thrust of the breathing which travels through the vertebral canal into the brain and expedites from there the formative forces— which you can get your hands on through the movements for vowels—you will be able to do this, if you have precisely such a case before you by having the child carry out the 'L'- movement. If you simply study eurythmy therapy, the way in which you should apply it will become clear to you through the diagnosis. Without a diagnosis it should not be practised, because in certain circumstances one can do entirely the wrong thing! However, it is indeed a fact that you have to awaken in yourself a feeling for the artistic element in the dynamics of the whole human being. Develop an intuitive eye for this artistic element.

Let us assume that the child is observed to experience certain difficulties at the time it begins to teethe; it has certain disorders which shouldn't be present. You discover that the intestinal movement is irregular and insufficient. With the 'L'-movement you are properly prepared. After the 'L'- movement has been carried out for a time, you assist what has been conducted to the sculptural centre with the move- ments for 'A' and 'O'. The vowel movements do affect the exhalation and already begin to work in the brain. The stream of breathing works in the brain. Everything associated with inhalation, in its most extensive, inclusive sense, is expressed in the consonantal element. This can be reinforced and promoted through consonantal eurythmy. Everything to do with exhalation can be reinforced by doing the vowels in eurythmy. When you do the vowels in eurythmy, however, the sculptural principle works directly together with the radiating principle—you have to decide how many times to repeat the sounds, how much energy is to be applied. Let us say, for example, we are faced with a kidney disturbance of one sort or another.[65] You may say to yourself that the kidney disturbance is at one stage or another, let's say in the initial stage. The moment that I have performed certain movements—for example, 'A'-movements*—I will have a beneficial effect on the kidney disturbance in its early stages. If the kidney disturbance has been present for a considerable time, and the insufficient function has already led to a deformation, I have first to prepare the ground with consonantal eurythmy followed by the vowels, in order to work on formation through the vowels as opposed to the deformation that has already taken place. In short, approach the matter as non-theoretically as possible; discover, solely out of knowledge of the human organism in its healthy and diseased states what was given in those rules I set out in Dornach and which have been passed on to you.

Now if, for example, it should be a case of a suppressed heart-lung function which in turn affects the kidneys, one will make progress in the initial stages with the movements for 'B' or 'P'. From this you will see that here one has the entire functioning in hand, and that everything depends upon one's understanding that a kind of centrifugal dynamic is present in each separate human organ, sculpturally rounded off by another dynamic working from without inwards—a dynamic that is not exactly centripetal, but which could be designated as similar to a centripetal dynamic that works into every human organ. We will only be able to pursue the study of physiology properly when we are able to contemplate each separate human organ in its polarity. These polarities, a centrifugal and a centripetal dynamic, lie within each human

---

* In another transcript 'S' appears here instead of 'A' (Ed. of 5th Germ. Edition, Dornach 2003).

organ. For everything that sculpts plays a significant role—the distribution and differentiation of the relative warmth in the human organism and the organization of the air conditions. For everything that is centrifugal, radiating, a great role is played by that which in the human organism comes from the dynamic of the substances of the world themselves, and what is developed in overcoming the inherent vitality of external nature in the human organism.[66] These two dynamics must be regulated reciprocally, and one can hope that eurythmy therapists will cultivate a fine feeling for what can be achieved in various instances. Precisely here extraordinarily much will depend upon an artistic disposition of the soul.

When you take into consideration that the whole system of eurythmy therapy can be reinforced by actual therapeutic methods, you find two factors working together. You can say to yourself, such and such affects the heart in particular in this or that way; you can reinforce that effect with a eurythmy therapy exercise. Then one thing will promote the other in a complementary manner. That is something which opens up truly great vistas, which can have an extraordinarily great future. Just think of the effect of massage, in some instances. I do not want to say anything against it or to criticize it; I acknowledge its importance. Yet this outward scratching about on the human being is inconsequential compared to the massage you apply when inducing entire systems of organs that work together to move inwardly in a different manner, through the elements of eurythmy therapy. That is the most inward kneading of the whole organism, affecting the etheric, the astral and the ego organisms. It is possible to say that what one recognizes as correct in massage is, in an endlessly powerful way, internalized through eurythmy therapy. One will in fact first gain an insight into the curative effects of gymnastics as well when one examines the resemblance between gymnastic exercises and eurythmical exercises. What is therapeutic in gymnastics is only of secondary importance to what is significant in eurythmy therapy. As I said at that time in Dornach, if you have the 'E'-movement carried out in a rhythmic sequence in the manner demonstrated, you do a great deal to help weak-looking children—children who only feebly carry through their bodily functions—to become more healthy and to begin to become stronger, as one would wish to see them. It is necessary, however, to take the whole human being into consideration in such matters. Again and again it happens that the entire human being is taken too little into consideration. I know that is a triviality, for you will say, 'Of course, we know that.' Indeed, but in practice it is repeatedly not taken into consideration. How often one hears: this person has an irregularly functioning heart, something must be done for it. Yes, but if one were to take the entire human being into consideration one would have to say, 'Thank God he has such a heart; his organism couldn't tolerate a normal one!' Similarly, under certain circumstances, one would have to say of a person who had broken his nose that he had suffered a favourable stroke of fate. If he breathed in air through completely developed channels, he would have too much air for his organism to process. What has its foundations in the organism as a whole must everywhere be taken into consideration.

When the movements for 'I' are carried out in a certain manner, they tend to harmonize the association of the right and the left sides of the human organism. With 'I' one can help in all asymmetries that appear in the human organism.

Through a cautious use of 'I'-movements you can produce excellent results with eurythmy therapy, even in the case of squinting. With squinting I would only advise that you do not proceed as you would with, for example, a person who walks asymmetrically, or who can use the right and left arms too asymmetrically. For squinting I would apply the usual 'I'-movements but would carry them out only with the index finger. In this way I would have them repeated as often as possible during the day. When the person is still growing this can bring good results, especially if the 'I' is carried out with the big toe as well. The best results, though, will be achieved when you can bring the patient to do it with the *little* toe as well. On the asymmetries affecting the sight these eurythmical exercises performed at the periphery will have a most beneficial effect. On the other hand, when it is a question of evening out a clumsiness in the manner in which a person walks, it could even bring good results to have him do the reverse, that is, to carry out the 'I'-movement with the line of vision, as when sighting—provided, of course, it does him no harm. In fact, one can really establish a sort of law—everything which is abnormal in the lower human being tends to be normalized by what is created as a compensation in the upper man, and vice versa.

When you find insecurities in standing, which may arise of course in the most varied manners, the forms of 'U' will be of especial importance. However, you must see that the 'U'-form is brought to completion so that the limbs concerned are really contiguous. This direct mutual contact, so that one limb feels the other, is of particular importance. Only then is the 'U'-form complete. In artistic eurythmy it is only necessary to indicate that this is so; in eurythmy therapy, however, it must be carried out. One limb is brought up against the other, so that you stand as 'at attention' with the legs pressed against one another. That is an extraordinarily therapeutic exercise for people who are affected with a compulsive twitching in the head. When it is fitting to treat corpulent children by means of eurythmy therapy, the 'O'-forms serve the purpose well. All these forms, if they are intended to bring results as eurythmy therapy, must be combined with a distinct perception of the muscular system involved. If you simply do the 'O'-form as many eurythmists do, it will suffice as an outward indication. It will not have a therapeutic effect, unless in the process of doing the exercise you feel the muscles throughout the arm. The slack swinging form has no effect; the sensation of the whole muscular system in its details, however, will bring the respective therapeutic-eurythmical result. It is particularly important to take heed that the eurythmy-therapy exercise is strengthened by extending it into the consciousness. When you do the 'O'-movement as I just did it, it is associated with a strong projection into the consciousness. Tell the fat one whom you treat with the 'O'-form: 'Think of your bigness, of your own girth, when doing the "O"!' In this way the consciousness centres on exactly that which is to be remedied. You reinforce in its innermost nature what is intended. The element of consciousness is not in the least to be under-estimated in healing.

In this connection, I have reason to believe that when these things become known, a battle with the orthopaedists will take place. Despite the fact that they are experiencing a great deal of success in their field at the present time, they are quite intent on viewing and treating the human being as a sort of mechanism. In the case of appliances used therapeutically so that the person in question should continually feel them, that they enter his awareness, this consciousness is an excellent remedial factor. Let us say, for example, that I find it would be advantageous for someone to straighten his shoulders, and I give him bandages which bring to his awareness that the shoulders should be held back—in other words, so that the treatment isn't carried out unconsciously. It is exactly the same in eurythmy therapy. These matters are brought to consciousness, in order that (as I have already said) this concentration vitally reinforce the process of therapeutic eurythmy itself.

I'd like to tell you something of particular importance. Everything that is an 'E'-form has a regulatory effect where the astral organism affects the etheric organism either too strongly or too weakly. In all those cases where you determine that either an exaggerated or an insufficient activity of the astral organism is present, then—other things being equal— you will be able to achieve a great deal with the 'E'-forms, with their repetition. 'E'-forms could have a therapeutic effect upon both complexes of symptoms which I described in the previous session.[67] What I have just said is particularly true when the astral organism is under the influence of the etheric, when it is too weak, when it permits itself to be influenced by the etheric, which itself is too strong as the result of an irregularity in the astral organism of the head. The opposite condition in which the etheric is too strongly affected by the astral may also arise. That would be the case when the astral comes very forcefully to expression in the intestine, when someone gets diarrhoea on every occasion when he is a bit afraid. Here the 'U'-forms will have an especially advantageous effect.

Yesterday a question arose which I would like to discuss briefly here, in closing. Can one allow persons who are pregnant or who have gynaecological complaints to do certain eurythmical movements? Just examine what was given as a rule in Dornach. You should be able to adhere to it even though in the case of pregnant women and gynaecological patients you must make certain that the abdomen is left in peace. It must be left undisturbed, must not be irritated by therapeutic eurythmy exercises. Although the abdomen itself is left in peace, and while that which must have quiet is in complete repose, exercises may nevertheless definitely be done with the arms while sitting, or while lying down, and with the head. You will still find enough in the indications given to be able to take measures through eurythmy therapy.

Naturally, when the person cannot move at all eurythmy would be quite the most beneficial for him, as in the case of paralytic symptoms; but under the circumstances the person cannot carry them out. They would definitely be the most wholesome. Such paralytic symptoms are of course in essence an abnormal functioning of the astral body, which does not engage itself in the etheric and physical organization. Here you will be able to achieve a great deal with 'E'-movements. An 'E'-movement that is very beneficial for disturbances of the abdomen is a carefully performed, not exaggerated, artificial crossing of the eyes. It is in fact true that the somewhat decadent yogis, who do certain exercises in which they focus their eyes on the tip of the nose, really intend to evoke the most harmonic activity of the abdomen possible, since they know the significance of abdominal activity for what such people call spiritual activity. One can say that matters are such that certain things that a person with a healthy abdomen would do with jumps can simply be replaced with a lighter eurythmy of the arms, the fingers, or even the eyes when it is necessary. A pregnant woman should never be induced to do eurythmy therapy exercises with jumps. That, of course, won't do.

As you see, it was not intended to produce a panacea that could be learnt in half a day. Eurythmy therapy too must be acquired through earnest labour, and it is necessary in fact that it is acquired through practice. For practically every time you practise a little, with your therapeutic instincts, therapeutic eurythmy exercises, you will be able to make better use of them. It is indeed so; through practice you will make exceptionally good progress, quite particularly in eurythmy therapy.

It was my intention to present you with this more theoretical discussion of eurythmy therapy, because everything else having to do with it—to the extent eurythmy therapy exists at present—was given earlier in Dornach and will be handed on by our physician friends, thus becoming available to you. And I wanted to give you the possibility of understanding the whole physiological and therapeutic meaning of eurythmy. Of course, on the other hand, one must not overestimate something like eurythmy therapy. In many cases it will be an extraordinarily important resource, but one should not overestimate it. One must make clear to oneself that really nothing can be achieved with 'intoxicating simplicity'. One can no more heal a broken leg or broken arm through therapeutic exercises alone than one can heal a carcinoma through the 'intoxicating simplicity of harmonizing the disharmonious'. One must be absolutely clear, an increase in dilettantism and medical amateurism is not to be found on the path of spiritual science, but rather a definite enrichment of professional medical ability. Excuse me for emphasizing it so often; in order to prevent misunderstandings, however, I particularly want to stress again that the methods are not brought forward in amateurish opposition to official medicine, as is often the case in fanatical movements. They take into account the state of medical science at present, and desire only to lead it along the path it has to be led, for the simple reason that it is not true that the human being is only that which the physiology and anatomy of today maintain. He is that, to be sure, but he is something more as well; he must be recognized from the aspect of his soul and spirit. Then those peculiar mental pictures that constantly show up nowadays, in which, for example, the brain is seen as a sort of central telegraphic apparatus to which the so-called sensory nerves run and from which the motor nerves lead, will disappear. The whole matter has no relation to reality, as will have become clear to you through today's lecture. In the nerve-sensory system we are dealing rather with a kind of sculptural dynamic, from which something is wrung which then accommodates itself to the activity of the soul. There is a great deal to be done in order to give back to a healthy physiology what has been taken from it through the correlations incorrectly established between the physical organism and the functions of the soul. Something physical is indeed present for every function of the soul during the course of human life on earth, but, on the other hand, nothing is used for the soul which has not a much greater importance for the bodily organization in its reciprocal action with the other organs. Nothing which is used for the soul is used merely as an organ of the soul. Our entire soul and spiritual make-up is wrested from the bodily nature, is taken out of the bodily nature. We may not permit ourselves to indicate certain organs as belonging to the soul. We could only say that the soul-functions are such that, disengaged from the organic functions, they are particularly adapted to the activity of the soul. Only when we become earnest about what is at work in the human organism, when, no longer proceeding in so outward a fashion, we picture the whole nervous system as an insertion serving the life of the soul, can we hope to perceive the human organization as it is. Only when the human organism is so perceived can it provide the basis for a physiology and therapy working in the light, not groping in the dark. I make this last remark to you, so that you yourselves do not leave here under a misunderstanding, and to enable you to counter misunderstandings which repeatedly arise.

Our carcinoma medication, for example, has been criticized with the 'intoxicating simplicity' that arises from people having no idea whatever about the knowledge through which the medication was derived. People have constructed instead some simple analogy or other and believe that, in disposing of the analogy, the matter itself can be done away. A proviso for the development and growth of the spiritual-scientific side of medicine is that one confront the misunderstandings, at least to a degree. People will soon notice that when they cannot spread misunderstandings they will have very little at all to say, for the principal concern of the opponents is the broadcasting of misconceptions about the whole of anthroposophy. Count how many adversaries have something other than misconceptions to relate. I must say that I often read antagonistic articles or essays and could connect them with something else entirely, were my name not present. It has no relation to what is nurtured here; it deals with something entirely different.

Sometimes I am very much surprised and would like to go and search out where what is being refuted has been expounded; in any case not here. In medicine the same thing is done as in theology; there one encounters it as well. One can, for example, say to a theologian at the pinnacle of his science that we have the same to say about Christ as you, only somewhat more. He is, however, not content when one says what he himself says, and then something in addition. He maintains one should not add anything to it. He does not criticize what is contrary to his assertions, he criticizes what he says nothing at all about. He criticizes what is said, simply because one speaks about something he knows nothing about. He considers it a mistake to claim to know something about which he himself knows nothing. Medicine must not fall into this error! We must observe accurately, and, rather than contradicting, we must add a great deal, out of an extremely well-founded knowledge of the healthy and diseased human being.

How Eurythmy Therapy *Came About, and its Significance*

Reports by Erna van Deventer-Wolfram, Elisabeth Baumann and Isabella de Jaager

Erna van Deventer-Wolfram★

Erna van Deventer, née Wolfram (1894–1976), eurythmist. One of the first pupils of eurythmy. Her interest in the therapeutic side of eurythmy led to Rudolf Steiner's decision to hold the lecture course, Eurythmy Therapy; *for decades she was active as a eurythmist and eurythmy therapist.*

I have two rather faded pieces of paper in front of me; one is a small drawing of the Cassinian curve and the other is a postcard dated February 1921, from Dr Roman Boos [the organizer at the time] in Dornach. Two modest pieces of paper, and yet they are almost the only visible testimonies of the events that led up to the eurythmy therapy lecture course that Dr Steiner gave in Dornach in the spring of 1921, alongside the second lecture course for doctors [GA 313].

If I want to go back in memory to the time when Dr Steiner gave the first eurythmy therapy exercises, I have to go much further back than 1921. As early as 1915 and even earlier, in answer to our questions Dr Steiner gave me—and probably

★ From 'Erinnerungen und Gedanken über den Weg der Enstehung der Heil-Eurythmie', in *Blätter für Anthroposophie*, ed. Hans Erhard Lauer, 13. Jg. Nr. 10, Basel 1961.

other eurythmy teachers, too—various eurythmy exercises for speaking, and hints for their use in the special cases we had encountered in towns all over Germany. The term *Heileurythmie* did not even exist then. Dr Steiner called these exercises *therapeutische* (therapeutic) eurythmy and said that these arose out of the Greek Mysteries. This remark will perhaps show how earnest he was even at that time about the art of healing by means of eurythmical movements. It will also show how deeply it was impressed upon the consciousness of us still very young teachers that *Heilung*, 'healing' is connected with *heil*, 'sacred, holy'; our movements in this eurythmy therapy would really have to be carried by 'the will to heal' if we wanted to achieve any success with this therapy. (Dr Steiner only later coined the expression 'the will to heal' in 1923–24, whereupon he entered into our problems and gave the lecture course for young medical students.)

Anyone who worked with Dr Steiner in any way will remember that everything he gave was in answer to a question, a wish, or sometimes even a vague aspiration that came his way. It was the same with eurythmy therapy. For example, two children with speech defects were brought to him, and he gave what we would later on have called 'eurythmy therapy exercises'. In 1919 I met a child with curvature of the spine. Dr Steiner entered into my questions very thoroughly and gave me the help I wanted. I could give many more examples like this. Yet at the same time I myself was also learning, in the course of giving lessons, to observe people, and I learnt to unite the various phenomena I observed in a person, and to become aware of how many people in the numerous eurythmy courses round about were in need of help...

During those years I often met Elisabeth Baumann-

Dollfus, who was also one of the first eurythmists. A deep love for the work we shared united us for many years. In 1919, after the end of World War I, we encountered one another again when the Waldorf School was being founded. So we began to exchange our experiences, she being a teacher at the Waldorf School where she worked with Dr Schubert's remedial class, and I being a eurythmist who in the course of the year gave eurythmy courses in almost all the big towns in Germany. I had the privilege when I was in Stuttgart of standing in for Frau Baumann at the Waldorf School when she was ill. We each had much joy in the other, because we were aware of our common bond. We were both searching for the same thing. This was the *healing element* in or behind eurythmy! This was one of the threads of destiny that bound us together. The other one was my engagement and marriage to H.A.R. van Deventer, himself a doctor. He approached eurythmy from a background of medicine with the same enthusiasm that we approached medicine from a background of eurythmy. And what gave rise to it? The lecture course on natural science given in Stuttgart during the Christmas season 1920/21.

Frau Baumann and I went to this lecture course, more as visitors really, since we could not understand very much of what Dr Steiner was saying, and as eurythmists we hardly even belonged to that enlightened gathering of students and scholars! But even if we did not understand it all with our intellects, our enthusiasm for the astronomical drawings made up for it.

One day, Dr Steiner drew something on the blackboard that made us nudge each other and nearly jump up, and that was the Cassinian curve. This was the *external* occurrence that we needed to make us aware that the paths of the stars and the flow of forces *within* us both sprang from the same source. For this curve of Cassini that Dr Steiner was now describing in connection with natural science and astronomy, why, we eurythmists knew it too! As early as 1915, in the White Room of the First Goetheanum, Dr Steiner had given four to six eurythmy teachers a series of lessons, and on this occasion he taught us 'children's forms, good for children and young people from the age of three to 80, to stop their thoughts getting scatty'. Those were his words, and one of these forms was the Cassinian curve, to the words, 'We want to seek one another; we feel each other near; we know each other well!'

In 1915, we young people did not have the least idea why he gave this form as an educational exercise, in fact we hardly knew the 'why' of any of the eurythmy teaching material— and, to be honest, do we know it that much better today? And yet it should be our task to pass on to our successors not only the exercises but also the 'why'. The only way to do this seems to be that in the eurythmy of the future we must separate truth from error, and the source of eurythmy from a watering-down of it.

This experience of 'recognizing' such an apparently insignificant form was what drew me to Elisabeth Baumann, and what caused her and my husband to sit together for hours discussing the problem. 'If this form which Dr Steiner was illustrating in the natural science lecture course is so important for both macrocosmic man and microcosmic man, then does not everything given us in eurythmy come from the same source, and should it not be applicable for therapy?' For just as with the Cassinian curve we had also over the years learnt about the *cosmic* and the *human* healing effect of vowels, for instance AUM. Our experience of the Cassinian curve was really only the cornerstone of the building of our surmises and experiences in the realm of eurythmy.

But how was it to be done? How were we to acquire a knowledge of 'eurythmy therapy'? What we knew up till then, Elizabeth Baumann and I, were only small building stones that on occasion Dr Steiner had given us. Through the fact that my husband, as a doctor, supported us in our ideas—he had done quite a lot of eurythmy himself, and could understand and support our endeavours from both the medical and the eurythmical side—this gave us courage to ask Dr Steiner, whilst he was still in Stuttgart, whether he would like to teach us a kind of eurythmy therapy in a systematic way just as he had taught us ordinary eurythmy. Dr Steiner was very kind, looked at us somewhat astonished at our bold plans, and said he would discuss the matter further with my husband in Holland, and then we would hear.

And thus it took place. Dr Steiner was in Holland at the beginning of 1921, and as my husband was strongly connected to our work through his medical studies he had a good deal of opportunity to talk with Dr Steiner. Frau Baumann was in Stuttgart at the time and I was in Breslau, but we had both set down our wishes very clearly in writing and sent them to my husband (still my fiancé at that time). At any rate, Dr Steiner asked him one day in Holland, 'Do you actually have some eurythmists who would really put their backs into eurythmy therapy?'—to which my husband replied, 'Yes indeed, two at present, Frau Baumann and my future wife.' 'Then we can start with that,' said Dr Steiner, and instructed my husband to do the necessary organizing. This brings me back to the beginning, for the little drawing was the 'Cassinian curve' which came from an evening's discussion with Dr Steiner, and the faded postcard from Roman Boos was his announcement from Dornach to say that the 'Eurythmy therapy lecture course' (Dr Steiner had now coined the name) was due to take place in Dornach at the beginning of April [GA 315], along with the second doctors' lecture course [GA 313], which was also due to be given then.

In an article,* Erna von Deventer-Wolfram describing how it was, writes: During the second doctors' course, from 12 to 17 April 1921 [GA 313], Dr Steiner gave the eurythmy therapy lecture course [GA 315] in six lectures, for doctors and also for eurythmists who had been training for more than two years. Not one of us could imagine what the lecture course would be like! Dr Steiner stood on the platform, and Frau Baumann and I, sitting on two chairs in front of it, felt very uncomfortable, for we had instigated the situation. In the meantime, from February till April, we had heard no word from Dr Steiner as to how he would establish this new branch of medical science with the likes of us, who had not the slightest preparatory training in the realm of medicine!

We certainly did not have the necessary knowledge for eurythmy therapy work. Would it not have been much more practical and sensible for Dr Steiner to have chosen a small group of doctors for this work? Or did Frau Baumann and I, being eurythmists, really bring something with us out of our past that seemed important to him? In the instructions he gave me shortly after the course, about the training necessary for eurythmy therapy, I received my answer.

He answered our questions by saying, 'The prerequisite for the profession of eurythmy therapist is that you first of all

---

* 'Heil-Eurythmie: 1921–71. Ihre Entstehung, Entwicklung und Aufgabe' in *Beiträge zu einer Erweiterung der Heilkunst nach Geisteswissenschaftlichen Erkenntnissen* (1971. Heft 4).

know the whole foundation of artistic eurythmy, in theory and practice. You must be capable of performing a dramatic poem on stage, for example Goethe's *Der Zauberlehrling* ('The Sorcerer's Apprentice'), and carry out all the eurythmical indications for the meaning of the words and the sentence construction, with all the forms and postures you have learnt. Not until you have mastered all the aspects of artistic eurythmy are you ready to change over to eurythmy therapy.'

He made it clear to us that we would first of all have to master all the possibilities of artistic eurythmy, be able to find them in the cosmos as the forces of the planets and the fixed stars, then in their reflection in human speech and music, then through movements of the human body itself, and in this way we would get to know the human being, that is, ourselves, as beings who reflect macrocosm and microcosm in our own body. Not until we had grasped our situation and task would we be able to advance from the periphery of eurythmy to the centre of the healing aspect of eurythmy. Yet 'first of all you must know the periphery, and then you can move on to the centre of man!' What a perspective for us, who had already been actively engaged in artistic and educational eurythmy for eight years, though more in a practical way, and by learning from doing it rather than filling it with our consciousness. The vowels, consonants, parts of speech, rhymes—how much more significant they now appeared to be!

...What a eurythmist should know was also clearly defined by Dr Steiner telling me what and how I would have to learn from my husband's textbooks, those by Prof. Spalteholz (Leipzig, February 1914) and Prof. Broesicke (Breslau, 1920).

Dr Steiner told us this shortly after the eurythmy therapy lecture course, so that it was with a deep feeling of responsibility that we took our departure from Dornach.

Elisabeth Baumann*

Elisabeth Baumann-Dollfus (1895–1947) actively participated in the development of eurythmy from the summer of 1913. Later she was the first eurythmy teacher at the Waldorf School, Stuttgart, founded in 1919. She was an active participant of the eurythmy therapy lecture course.

Children of all ages grasped and carried out the movements of eurythmy so naturally that we experienced every day of our lives that the visible, movement-language of eurythmy is a language that is in genuine harmony with the laws and requirements of both man's spiritual and soul nature and his bodily nature. We also experienced daily that hindrances the children had, whether in the realm of the will or in the realm of mental picturing, of the activity of thinking, could be loosened up or actually overcome by eurythmy. At the Waldorf School almost from the very beginning we had to deal with children who had hindrances of this sort. Sometimes these difficulties were only slightly in evidence; sometimes the children were so overwhelmed by them that they could not keep up with the lessons of their class. A special remedial class was started where they could be given what Rudolf Steiner prescribed for their care.

---

*From the Foreword to the 1952 German edition of *Heileurythmie* (pp. vii–ix).

Experience showed that for children of this sort eurythmy more than anything else could get across to them and they could take immediate hold of it. Consequently, we asked ourselves whether it would be possible to find exercises that would help the spiritual part that was experiencing such difficulty in incarnating because it met with such strong bodily resistance. These exercises would give the physical sheath a better form—movement exercises that would help the etheric formative forces to penetrate better and give their support to the creative up-building forces of the organism.

Out of our close connection with difficult cases, with those in need of special care, we acquired the most intense desire to discover and take hold of the healthy, therapeutic element of eurythmy. From many conversations with Erna van Deventer-Wolfram, who was actively engaged in eurythmy in various parts of Germany, it transpired that through the work she was doing she, too, had been powerfully drawn to this therapeutic aspect of eurythmy.

After due reflection, we decided to ask Dr Steiner for instructions on eurythmy therapy. Rudolf Steiner agreed with alacrity and promised to think about it. It was not long before Frau van Deventer and I were requested to go to Dornach in April where he wanted to give lectures on eurythmy therapy [GA 315] alongside the doctors' lecture course [GA 313] he was going to give at the Goetheanum.

So it was during the days of 12 to 17 April 1921 that Rudolf Steiner presented the gift of the third element of eurythmy, and the doctors and eurythmists who were present experienced a whole new world of possibilities for therapy opening up before them. In its variety and effectiveness and the way in which Rudolf Steiner presented it, this was bound to have made an unforgettable impression on them. Instead of the few instructions and indications we had asked for, we were given a complete and detailed method of eurythmy therapy, in which we could directly experience that even today the creative and therapeutic power of the word, with its capacity to take hold of the movement potential in the human body, is still at work. It often happened that it was not easy to find our way into it, for even those of us who for many years had been familiar with the eurythmical art of movement found that the exercises Rudolf Steiner either carried out himself or asked Frau van Deventer-Wolfram and myself to carry out were utterly new and surprising. It was especially difficult for the doctors present, as only a minority had had anything to do with eurythmy up till then. Two eurythmy courses were set up to practise basic eurythmy with the doctors, and also the exercises that had been given by Dr Steiner during the eurythmy therapy lecture that day. Regular work at eurythmy therapy now started up in various places. In the clinics in Arlesheim and Stuttgart and also at the Waldorf School, Stuttgart, Rudolf Steiner gave several more indications for the use of eurythmy therapy in special cases. He himself varied the one or the other exercise, and he gave certain sound sequences that were to be practised with individual patients under his special observation. These indications offer doctors and eurythmy therapists a rich opportunity to learn more about a methodical approach, adapting of exercises to the individual needs of patients, and the scrupulous observation required for this.

The real basis of all eurythmy therapy work is given in this lecture course [GA 315], as is clearly stated in Rudolf Steiner's own words. In October 1922, on the occasion of a medical week in Stuttgart, he was again asked to speak about eurythmy therapy, this time by doctors. That lecture is included here with the 1921 course. Right at the beginning Rudolf Steiner says, 'The wish has been expressed for me to expound somewhat further upon eurythmy therapy. Basic-ally, the empirical material relating to eurythmy therapy was developed and presented in the recent lecture course for physicians in Dornach [GA 313], and it is hardly necessary to go beyond what was given at that time. Used in the proper manner, it will be of far-reaching importance.'

Isabella de Jaager*

Isabella de Jaager (1892–1979), eurythmist and eurythmy therapist, from 1928 Leader of the Eurythmy School at the Goetheanum. Founding member of the Rudolf Steiner Nachlass-verwaltung (R. Steiner's literary estate); editor of the 2nd German edition of Eurythmy Therapy *[GA 315] and the 2nd German edition (Dornach 1955) of* Eurythmy as Visible Speech *[GA 279].*

It will soon be evident to the reader that without a thorough study of anthroposophy you will not get very far with this eurythmy therapy lecture course [GA 315]. Eurythmy ther-apy arises out of anthroposophy just the same as artistic eurythmy does. A living grasp of man and the world is a necessary basis for its use. Only on this assumption will it avoid becoming a system or something that is grasped and applied in an abstract, intellectual way—an ever-present danger in our times. Eurythmy therapy also requires an

---

* Epilogue by I. de Jaager to the 1952 German edition of *Heileurythmie* (p. 107f.).

extensive knowledge of artistic eurythmy. Imaginative forces, the coming-into-movement of man's whole being, are prerequisites for the application of this therapy, where it is essential to have an artistic understanding of the patient. All the delicate and minute nuances needed in order to help a sick child or adult come to us out of artistic eurythmy. You will continually find new inspiration here.

I would like to stress that a young person should not devote him/herself exclusively to eurythmy therapy. Up to the age of 28 a person should be able to give his/her imagination and creative forces free rein. The more this can happen, the better he/she will be able to develop devotion, patience and empathy when doing eurythmy therapy later. It is essential to devote oneself wholly to the patient and carry him/her with artistic warmth of heart.

As Rudolf Steiner often mentions in the lecture course, eurythmy therapy should never be used without a doctor's thorough diagnosis. The greater the collaboration with the patient's doctor the more effective the eurythmy therapy will be.

Background to the Text and Drawings

The text

The six lectures on eurythmy therapy were taken down in shorthand by the professional stenographer Helene Finckh (1883–1960), who then wrote them out in longhand. Lecture 7, held during the 'Medical Week' in Stuttgart, was recorded by an unknown stenographer, who also wrote it out in longhand. Here the original shorthand report no longer exists.

These reports were gone over in detail for the earlier German editions. For the 5th edition, both the shorthand and longhand reports were again studied from beginning to end. After Michael Schweizer, Michaelis Messmer in collaboration with Dr med. Wilburg Keller Ruth and Walter Kugler undertook this word-for-word checking. The notes were extended, other appendices added, and the vote of thanks from Dr med. Friedrich Husemann included.

The drawings

The originals of the eurythmy therapy lecture course, drawn on grey card, still exist. After the lecture they were dated, fixed and saved. Reproductions are published in the collected works, Vol. XII of the series 'Wandtafelzeichnungen zum Vortragswerk' (K 58/22). Earlier editions contained good copies of the originals by Assya Turgeniev and Hedwig Frey; those of Lectures 5 and 7 originate from sketches of the blackboard drawings by the shorthand reporter. The artwork was undertaken by Priska Clerc. The original blackboard drawings no longer exist for the lecture held on 28 October, 1922 in Stuttgart.

Notes

Based on those of the 5th German edition, 2003,
with additions

List of publishers, etc., by abbreviation, mentioned in the notes

AP—Anthroposophic Press, Spring Valley, New York
AN—Anastasi Ltd., Weobley, UK
AP—Anthroposophic Press, Hudson, USA
APC—Anthroposophical Publishing Company, London, UK
CP—Completion Press, Gympie, Australia
MH—College of Teachers, Michael Hall School, Forest Row, UK
MP—Mercury Press, Spring Valley, USA
RSP—Rudolf Steiner Press, London, UK
SB—Sophia Books, an imprint of RSP
SBC—Steiner Book Centre, North Vancouver, Canada
SSF—Steiner Schools Fellowship Publications, Forest Row, UK
Typ—Typescript, Rudolf Steiner House Library, London, UK

Volumes from Rudolf Steiner's Collected Works mentioned in the notes, which are in English translation (ET)

GA 1   *Goethean Science*, MP, 1988
GA 5   *Friedrich Nietzsche, Fighter for Freedom*, Spiritual Science
          Library, Garber Communications, Inc., Blauvent, New
          York 1985
GA 10   *How to Know Higher Worlds*, AP, 1994
GA 13   *An Outline of Esoteric Science*, AP, 1997
GA 15   *Spiritual Guidance of the Individual and Humanity*, AP,
          1991

GA 18   *Riddles of Philosophy*, AP, 1973

GA 27   (R. S. & Ita Wegman) *Extending Practical Medicine*, RSP, 1996

GA 58   *Metamorphoses of the Soul*, Vol 1, RSP, 1983

GA 59   *Metamorphoses of the Soul*, Vol 2, RSP, 1983

GA 122   *Genesis*, RSP, 2002

GA 124   *Background to the Gospel of St Mark*, RSP, 1968

GA 130   *Faith, Love and Hope*, SBC, 1964

GA 134   *The World of the Senses and the World of the Spirit*, SBC, 1979

GA 174   *Karma of Untruthfulness*, Vol 2, RSP, 1992

GA 194   *The Archangel Michael: His Mission and Ours*, AP, 1994

GA 199   *Spiritual Science as a Foundation for Social Forms*, AP, 1986

GA 208   *Cosmosophy*, Vol 2, Completion Press, 1997

GA 209   *The Alphabet*, MP, 1982

GA 212   *The Human Soul in Relation to World Evolution*, AP, 1985

GA 218   *Spiritual Relations in the Human Organism*, MP, 1984

GA 230   *Harmony of the Creative Word*, RSP, 2001

GA 267   Selections in ET to be found in three vols, *Breathing the Spirit, Finding the Greater Self, Living with the Dead*, SB, 2002

GA 277   *Eurythmie—Der Offenbarung der Sprechenden Seele*, Dornach 1999

GA 277a *Eurythmy: Its birth and development*, AN, 2002

GA 278   *Eurythmy as Visible Singing*, Stourbridge 1998. Dist. <*eurythmy.wm@ukonline.co.uk*>

GA 279   *Eurythmy as Visible Speech*, AN, 2005

GA 280   *Creative Speech—The Nature of Speech Formation*, RSP, 1978

GA 282   *Speech and Drama*, APC, 1959, reprinted AP, 1986

GA 284   *Occult Seals and Signs*, Typ. date unknown, pt tr. RSE221 in RSH Library

GA 292   *Kunstgeschichte als Abbild innerer geistiger Impulse*, 2 vols,

Dornach 1981. History of Art. (Typ. date unknown. R11 in RSH Library)

GA 293   *Study of Man*, RSP, 1966/*Fundamentals of Human Experience*, AP, 1996

GA 300b *Faculty Meetings with Rudolf Steiner*, AP, 1998

GA 302a *Spiritual Knowledge as the Fount of Educational Art* ('Meditatively Acquired Knowledge of Man'), SSF, 1982

GA 303   *Soul Economy and Waldorf Education*, AP, 1986

GA 307   *Modern Art of Education*, RSP, 1972

GA 312   *Introducing Anthroposophical Medicine*, AP, 1999

GA 313   *Anthroposophical Spiritual Science and Medical Therapy*, MP, 1991

GA 314   *Fundamentals of Anthroposophical Medicine*, MP, 1986

GA 316   *Course for Young Doctors*, MP, 1994

GA 317   *Education for Special Needs*, RSP, 1998

GA 318   *Broken Vessels: The Spiritual Structure of Human Frailty*, SB, 2006

GA 324a *Fourth Dimension*, AP, 2001

NB: This is a developing field. For further and latest information, including many lectures available on-line, see <*www.rudolfsteinerweb.com*> and Rudolf Steiner Archive: <*www7.rsarchive.org*>, and Rudolf Steiner Libraries *http://rslibrary.elib.com* and *rsh-library@anth.org.uk*

In the following notes, translations of the quotations have been freshly made, with references to the published versions (where known) added in brackets.

Lecture 1

1. See the account of the beginnings in GA 277a, the two basic lecture courses on eurythmy, GA 278 and GA 279 (containing commentaries by A.S.), and the collection of introductions in GA 277. For a selection of 16 introductions from GA 277 in ET, see: *An Introduction to Eurythmy*, AP, 1984.

2. See, e.g., the introduction of 2 June 1918 in GA 277, ET p. 24. See also the lecture of 21 May 1907 in GA 284: 'The forces in us are condensed divine forces. What was created earlier by the Word is now transformed into natural forms. During the course of evolution the human larynx will become the organ of reproduction... What today is the organ of speech will become the producer of its own kind. The larynx is the future organ of reproduction raised into spirituality; with men already now the larynx develops parallel to the development/maturity of the sexual organs.' See also Armin J. Husemann, *The Harmony of the Human Body*, Floris Books, Edinburgh 2002, section 32.

3. During the lecture course running parallel at the time, R. Steiner spoke on 16 April 1921 about the metamorphoses of various organs, e.g., the lungs as 'a metamorphosis of the form of the head' GA 313 (ET p. 81). Further examples, see GA 293, especially Lecture 10. For basic concepts, see GA 1, Chapter 2.

See also R. Steiner's eurythmy form to Goethe's poem *Die Metamorphose der Pflanzen* in *Eurythmieformen*, Vol. 3, 'Eurythmieformen zu Dichtungen von Johann Wolfgang von Goethe', GA K23/3, Dornach 1990, pp. 41–52.

The concept is explained in detail in Kürschner's prestigious edition of Goethe's scientific works, ed. R. Steiner, 5 vols (1884–97); reprinted Dornach 1975, GA 1a–1e. In GA 1a, 'The Metamorphosis of the Plant', XVIII, 115, we read: 'The plant may sprout, blossom and produce fruit, but they are still *the same organs* which in many and various manifestations and under often most changed form fulfils the law of nature. The same organ, which extends itself on the twig as the leaf taking on most varied shapes, retracts in the chalice, extends itself again in the petals of the flower, contracts into the instruments of reproduction, finally expanding as a fruit.'

4. See also the lecture of 28 February 1911 in GA 124. Amongst

other things, we read: 'The participation, the living interest in things, is undermined when the thyroid is removed. People become listless to such an extent that they are not able to use their intellect. There you have the fine difference between the use of an instrument for the understanding, as it is part of the brain, and a tool having to do with the glands, as it is the thyroid gland' (ET p. 125).

5. See lecture of 21 April 1920 in GA 302a (ET p. 25). Basic facts about the development of the larynx are to be found in GA 15. See also note 2.

6. On the connection of head and rhythm, see lecture of 28 December 1921 in GA 303 (ET p. 85); lecture of 15 January 1917 in GA 174 (2nd Germ. ed. 1983, p. 150f.: ET p. 110).

7. Elisabeth Baumann reports: 'Two eurythmy courses were set up to practise basic eurythmy with the doctors, and also the exercises that had been given by Dr Steiner during the eurythmy therapy lecture that day.' See p. 135 in the present volume.

8. On the initiative of Emil Molt, Director of the Waldorf-Astoria cigarette factory, a comprehensive primary and secondary school was founded in autumn 1919 in Stuttgart for the children of the factory workers, but open to other children. Steiner took on working through a future-orientated concept of education as well as the choice and training of the teachers. Already in 1884 he demanded the freeing of education from every governmental prescription. In 1907 in his booklet *Die Erziehung des Kindes von Geschictspunkte der Geisteswissenschaft* (*The Education of the Child in the Light of Spiritual Science*), he stated the basic concept of man for a pedagogy and art of education orientated towards development. Prior to the founding of the school and during the years—till his death in 1925 he was the Principal of the Waldorf School—Steiner held numerous training courses for teachers as well as an abundance of lectures for parents, teachers and pupils at home and

abroad. Within the Collected Works, these were published in more than 20 volumes (GA 293–311). A help to approach Steiner/Waldorf education is the second volume of the series 'Quellentexte für die Wissenschaften', *Texte zur Pädagogik. Anthroposophie und Erziehungswissenschaft*, Rudolf Steiner Verlag, Dornach 2003, ed. by Johannes Kiersch.

In the Waldorf School, Stuttgart—the starting point for many further schools worldwide—eurythmy was an obligatory subject.

9. Further on this, see lecture of 11 November 1923 in GA 230 (7th Germ. ed. 1993, p. 205; ET p. 199).

10. Concerning geometrical figures, see Lecture 3 of GA 293 (ET p. 63). On writing with the feet, see GA 317 (Germ. ed. p. 147f.; ET p. 170): 'In such cases, and this is also a kind of eurythmy therapy, if he learns to write with the toes, eurythmy can be of great service.' See further GA 277a, p. 20.

11. See Lecture 4 of the parallel-running lecture course for doctors, GA 313 (ET p. 54).

12. On this, see Answers to Questions of 11 March 1920 in GA 324a (ET p. 117).

Lecture 2

13. Steiner spoke on the vowels and consonants expressing various soul-moods already in 1911 in his book GA 15 (ET p. 36ff.): 'In Atlantean times human beings felt all external impressions in such a way that the soul, when it wanted to express outer things with a speech sound, was impelled to use a consonant... What was inwardly experienced as pain or joy, or also what another being could feel, that one could imitate in a vowel.' A development of what is presented here is found in the lecture of 18 December 1921 in GA 209 (2nd Germ. ed., 1982, p. 110ff.; ET p. 8ff.).

14. See lecture of 9 January 1924 in GA 316 (3rd Germ. ed. 1987,

p. 133f.; ET p. 115), concerning amongst other things exercises for children inclined to stutter.

15. Migraines are fully discussed in lecture of 5 April 1920 in GA 312 (7th Germ. ed. 1999, p. 300f.; ET p. 222) and GA 27, chapter 20 (7th Germ. ed., p. 128f.; ET p. 113).
16. See GA 277a, p. 26. The sketch (p. 25) corresponds exactly to the one here.

Lecture 3

17. R. Steiner gave almost 300 introductions to eurythmy performances, some of which cover the basics of eurythmy, other individual details (formation of the sounds, individual organs, the limbs, relationship to the dance or mime, relationship to sculpture and architecture). A selection is published in GA 277; some are included in GA 277a. For a further selection in ET, see note 1.
18. Rudolf Steiner, *Riddles of Philosophy* (GA 18), AP, 1973. Originally a two-volume work (1900/01), expanded (1914) with a prolegomena on western philosophy to the time of writing.
19. Further points are to be found in the lecture of 2 July 1923 in GA 279, Lecture 7, ET p. 83. Additionally: GA 280, ET p. 89; GA 282, ET p. 61; GA 122 p. 22.
20. Further on this see GA 280 (ET p. 79) and GA 282, Lecture 18 (ET p. 379). Also GA 307, lectures of 8, 9 and 10 August 1923 (ET pp. 88, 105). See also Agatha Lorenz-Poschmann, *Die Sprachwerkzeuge und ihre Laute*, Philosophisch Anthroposophischer Verlag, Dornach 1983.
21. See GA 312, Lecture 11 (Germ. 7th ed. 1999, p. 216; ET p. 157).
22. See GA 293, Lecture 10 (Germ. 9th ed. 1992, p. 146f.; ET p. 159), and the discussion during the Faculty Meeting in GA 277a, p. 140; also the descriptions in GA 316 (Germ. ed. 1987, pp. 174 and 231; ET pp. 157 and 124). See too the

lecture of 30 June in GA 317 (Germ. 8th ed. 1995, p. 77; ET p. 89).

23. See GA 13, Chapter 4; also GA 218, Lectures 1 and 2.

Lecture 4

24. Emil Abderhalden (1877–1950), Swiss physiologist and physiological chemist. From 1911 to 1945 professor at the University of Halle a. d. Saale. Editor of *Handbuch der biologischen Arbeitsmethoden*. Basic works on social hygiene and social physiology. Concerning his stay in Dornach and his statements about teaching gymnastics, which R. Steiner refers to in other lectures, no further details are known.

25. See introductions to eurythmy performances of 17 October 1920 and 19 November 1920 in GA 277, 3rd ed., pp. 195 and 207. Concerning the relationship of gymnastics to eurythmy, Steiner speaks at length in the lecture of 13 June 1921, in GA 302 (Germ. 5th ed., p. 38ff.; ET p. 7).

Lecture 5

26. See lecture 'The Sun Mystery in the Course of Human History', 6 November 1921 in GA 208 (3rd Germ. ed. p. 166ff.; ET p. 171), RSP, 1955, and basics in GA 293, Lecture 5 (ET p. 95).

27. See lecture 'Faith, Love and Hope: three stages of human life' in GA 130.

28. See note 15.

29. On this see the lecture of 6 July 1924 in GA 317 (8th Germ. ed. p. 97; ET p. 189). See also GA 277a, p. 31.

30. Rudolf Steiner spoke at length about laughing (and crying) in the Architektenhaus in Berlin, public lecture of 3 February 1910, in GA 59.

31. R. Steiner spoke of the task, meaning and significance of the feeling of devotion in his book *Knowledge of the Higher Worlds—how is it achieved?*, GA 10, Chapter 1. See lecture of 28 October 1909, 'The Mission of Devotion', in *Metamor-*

phoses of the Soul, Part 1, GA 58; also the lecture of 17 February 1910, 'The Essence of Prayer', in *Metamorphoses of the Soul,* Part 2, GA 59.

32. In his address on the occasion of the first eurythmy performance in Munich, 28 August 1913, Steiner relates that the human etheric body should dance. See GA 277a, p. 52.

33. On gymnastics, see the Conference of the Waldorf School, 1 March 1923, in GA 300b (Germ. ed. 1975, p. 292ff.; ET p. 570). See also note 24.

34. In Lecture 3, where the lecturer speaks of the connection of the sound-creations ('O' and 'E') and the human organism.

35. *Der Ablauf des Lebens. Grundlegung zur exakten Biologie,* Leipzig and Vienna 1906. In the chapter on left-handedness (pp. 439–41), we read: 'Observers have completely overlooked the main thing, that with left-handed men the secondary female sexual character and with left-handed women the secondary male sexual character is much more predominant than by right-handed males and females. If you ask a man, for example, an artist who through his whole type belongs to the "realm between", that is, contains much femininity, if he is left-handed, you first receive the answer "Not at all", he bears no trace of it. In his own way, he is right, since he does not know of these things, and a dim feeling determines people to deny left-handedness. *Linkisch* (gausche) has the other meaning of "not quite complete". But looking at both of his hands, one can often see that the right hand does not predominate, rather the left hand is the same size but perhaps even more strongly developed. This is sometimes especially shown by the position of the thumb.' Wilhelm Fließ (1858–1928) was a throat, nose and ear physician and biologist in Berlin. He was known through his teaching on the periodicity of life, and his relationship to Sigmund Freud. The letters of Freud to Fließ are regarded as important historical documents in the development of psychoanalysis.

36. See both lectures of 18 April: the morning lecture in GA 313; and the afternoon lecture, Lecture 7 in the present volume.

Lecture 6

37. Goethe's poem carries the title *Wanderers Nachtlied II* (The Wayfarer's Night Song II). Steiner also discusses this poem in *Eurythmy as Visible Singing*, GA 278, and *Eurythmy as Visible Speech*, GA 279. The translation by Longfellow is given in the notes to the ET of GA 278 ('Companion', p. 44); trs. by Henry W. Nevinson (*Goethe: Man and poet*, Nisbet, London 1931) and David Luke (*Johann Wolfgang von Goethe: Selected poetry*, Libris, London 1999) are included in the text of GA 279 (Lecture 8, p. 97).

38. Frau Dr Steiner, née Marie von Sivers (Wlotzlawek, Russia 1867–1948 Beatenberg, Switzerland). Studied recitation and acting in Saint Petersburg and Paris. Since 1902 close co-worker of Rudolf Steiner. She was first and foremost involved in building up the Anthroposophical Society, the development of eurythmy, the art of acting and speech formation at the Goetheanum and of the Philosophisch-Anthroposophischen Verlag. Alongside this she translated into German, among other works, some titles by Edouard Schuré.

39. See lecture of 18 April 1921, Lecture 7 in the present volume, p. 100: 'Listen carefully, bring intensely into consciousness the sound that you hear, the relationships of the sentence you hear, to which you are doing eurythmy.'

40. See GA 27, Chapter 1 (Germ. 7th ed. p. 12; ET p. 6): 'It is of the greatest importance to know that the normal forces of human thinking are the most refined forces of form and growth. In the form and growth of the human organism a spiritual [entity] is revealed. This appears in the course of life as the spiritual force of thinking.' See also GA 312, ET p. 244.

41. See Lecture 6 of the parallel-held doctors' lecture course GA 313.

42. See too the parallel-held doctors' lecture course GA 313, and Lectures 16 and 18 of GA 312.

43. See on this Lecture 2 of the parallel-held doctors' lecture course GA 313 (Germ. ed. p. 49; ET p. 49): 'For in part, at least for the system of the head and breathing, the "I" and astral body separate themselves completely from the physical body and ether body—not for the human being of digestion and of the circulation, in them they remain. It is not exact to say that the "I" and astral body depart. It is actually correct to say—and here I have earlier, for many years now, frequently indicated this—in sleep for the organization of the head, "I" and astral body leave the physical body and ether body, but in the organization of digestion and of the circulation they penetrate it all the more.'

44. See the lectures of 22 and 23 April 1924 in GA 316.

45. Steiner overviews this theme out of his experience as a home tutor and educator in the lecture of 1 July 1924 in GA 317 (Germ. 8th ed. 1995, p. 95f.; ET p. 110).

46. See Lecture 4 of the parallel-held doctors' lecture-course GA 313.

47. On the connection between the human being and the cosmos through the rhythm of breathing and of sleep, see GA 312 (Germ. ed. p. 126f.; ET p. 90): 'The movements of the heart are not only an impression of that which occurs in the human being, but absolutely an impression of relationships beyond the human being.'

48. See the lectures of 19 and 20 November 1922 in GA 218. See also note 44.

49. A form of medical gymnastics devised by the Swedish poet Peter Henry Ling (1776–1839). When gymnastics in the 18th century in various European countries became by and by a stable part of education, people initially inclined to the ideals of the ancient Greeks. That is why the word 'gymnastics' was used. And so one speaks of a Swedish 'medical gymnastics',

which distinguished three basic kinds of movement: the active movement, where the patient mostly in a lying position, carries out the movement alone; the semi-active or duplicating movement, where, to the movements of the patient through a second person, a stronger or weaker resistance is given; finally, the passive movement, not carried out by the patient, which the therapist carries out on the body of the patient and which is mostly connected with kneading, knocking or caressing manipulations (massage). See P.H. Ling, *Allgemeine Begründung der Gymnastik* (1840); Dr Ander Wide, MD, *Handbook of Medical Gymnastics* (1899).

50. Eurythmy was an obligatory subject in the Waldorf School, Stuttgart. See note 8.

51. Dr med. Friedrich Husemann (1887–1959), psychiatrist. Member of the Theosophical Society and Anthroposophical Society since 1910. From 1921 to 1924 doctor at the Klinisch-Therapeutischen Institut in Stuttgart. In 1925 he founded a Sanatorium in Freiburg-Günterstal, which moved in 1930 to Wiesneck.

Lecture 7

52. See lecture of 26 March 1920 in GA 312.

53. See lectures of 1, 5 and 6 April 1920 in GA 313.

54. Described in detail in lecture of 23 April 1920 in GA 316.

55. Earlier editions read *durchströmen* (stream through); the shorthand can also be read as *Durchträumen* (dream through). The later reading could be preferable, since Steiner refers in this sentence to 'yesterday's lecture' [i.e., Lecture 6], where a similar connection between a kind of sleeping and dreaming is discussed.

56. Mechthild von Magdeburg (*c.* 1207–82) the first known female mystic to write in German. She grew up in a well-to-do family, took up in 1230 the ascetic life in Marburg after her first deep divine experience at 12 years old. About 1270 she

moved to Kloster Helfta and completed her most important work, begun in 1250, *Ein fließendes Licht der Gottheit*, in which she criticized the riches of some clerics and of the cathedral centre, bringing on herself great difficulties. One of her most well-known poems from the above-mentioned work is *Ich kann nicht tanzen, o Lord, es sei denn sie führen mich* (I cannot dance, O Lord, unless it be they lead me). See Steiner's comments in GA 318 (ET p. 57).

57. Theresa of Avila (1515–82), Spanish mystic and Carmelite. Her teaching of completion, of the mystic marriage with God, is recorded in several writings. In close collaboration with St John of the Cross (1542–91), she reformed under great difficulties the Carmelite order. She was raised to sainthood in 1622. See Steiner's comments in GA 318.

[In the text, the few editorial additions within square brackets attempt to elucidate this obscure passage, touching on the most stubborn traits of the human condition, art and the healing process. The fact that two mystics are brought into the discussion here in connection with personal matters suggests something important is addressed—moreover, the advice is given in non-moralistic language. Earlier in his lecturing career, e.g., in GA 134 (1911) which can provide a context here, Steiner speaks of a pre-lapsarian humanity. Humanity entered more deeply into incarnation than was planned by the spiritual world. Steiner faces the origin of evil, death and illness and the long-term counter-remedy. He describes what the biblical account terms paradisaical existence; in this lecture course details are given of the divine redemptive healing power which counteracts the Fall of man, otherwise termed 'original sin', the congenital racial condition.

The comment in the text about the 'beautiful historical process' that includes drawing seems to affirm a sound interest in the earth. The 'reverse process', a *schwülen Dichtungen* (sultry/oppressive poetry), suggests an other-worldly mysticism. Steiner seems to be saying that what is often called a naturalistic tendency in art is a justified phase. It serves as the essential point of departure, or reference, for all later developments attempting to supersede the historical onlooker stage. This reading takes Steiner's *abstrakt* here to refer to human consciousness (not, for example, to a category of 20th-century art). The great artists of the Renaissance and onwards certainly achieved much more than mere naturalism, as Steiner often points out, for example, in his wide-ranging lectures on spiritual impulses in the history of art (GA 292). What is usually termed 'naturalism' is just one outcome—not only in art—of the onlooker attitude, or what Steiner terms the 'consciousness soul'. Upon this grounded basis, however, *all* sound human spiritual development of the future is built, summed up in the words 'scientific attitude' and 'self-knowledge'.

In the text here, the eurythmical example of a 'process of healing'—correcting unconscious, and probably questionable, escapist indulging—involves attention to the details of 'the sound that you hear, the relationships of the sentence you hear'. The alphabet of 'vowels and consonants'—generally regarded as merely abstract, since one symbol represents one sound—and indeed grammar, too, only appear as lifeless things. The alphabet can actually lead to the 'objective intuiting powers'. The abstract stage provides the technical means, the essential mirror for self-consciousness. The divine-human alphabet, the 'lost word' of occult tradition, reflects our complete human nature. (Lecture Dornach, 18 December 1921, GA 209; lecture Dornach, 24 June 1924, GA 279. Also note 12.) The experiential path uniting science, art and therapy here is revealed as the teacher exploring 'what is'—the creative Word itself reconstitutes its own image.

Regarding the references to the two mystical writers, it should be acknowledged that probably the most far-reaching image in the New Testament, marriage, connects the supreme redemptive deed of Good Friday (the Last Supper is a marriage feast) and the descent of New Jerusalem ('Jupiter-existence' in Steiner's terminology) 'adorned like a bride' (Rev. 21:2). Now, the 'human being of sense, glands and digestion', Steiner points out (GA 134), is a relic of the past. (Papageno, the Bird-Catcher of *The Magic Flute*, as Natural Man, might have a word to say here! To his credit it must be admitted that Papageno did find the captive Princess Pamina before his master Prince Tamino. In the language of fairy tales, however, this simply pictures the way of it; all the characters of a fairy tale present aspects of the whole human being.)

The nature of human blood is also discussed. Then, Steiner continues, what of human Imagination, Inspiration and Intuition is morally good and beautiful, arising from 'the human being of bone, muscle and nerve', is accepted by the spiritual world to form the new planetary embodiment. Redemption, marriage-union, is of the human race. We lead a communal life.

Daunting and challenging as the subject certainly is, yet at the same time it is hardly possible to suggest anything more authentic, beautiful and inspiring. By formulating the challenge of transformation as Steiner does—'getting your hands on', as he puts it in this present Lecture 8—already initiates a (or the) method of spiritual science, joining all related efforts that go beyond what could merely remain as a doctrine, an aspiration, a caricature or cheap nostrum. I can know that this act of mine which I now utter is to succeed and hold its place in history. 'This is apocalypse,' writes the very great literary critic Northrop Frye (1912–91), 'the complete transformation of both nature and human nature into the same form.' Our earth-existence is awaiting the change. Steiner's gift of *The Soul's Calendar* (1911) artistically explores this theme. (Note by A.S.)]

58. See also Lectures 1 and 2 in GA 317. Numerous further statements by Steiner on heredity can be found through the help of *Register zur Rudolf Steiner Gesamtausgabe*, Vol. A–L, under the entry 'Anthropologie', sub-entry 'Vererbung'.

59. Friedrich Nietzsche (1844–1900), German philosopher. His book *Jenseits von Gut und Böse: Vorspiel einer Philosophie der Zukunft* (*Beyond Good and Evil: Prelude to a philosophy of the future*) (1885/6), 'takes up and expands on the ideas of Nietzsche's previous work, *Thus Spoke Zarathustra*, replacing that work's sunny and life-affirming character with a highly critical, polemical approach. In *Beyond Good and Evil*, Nietzsche attacks past philosophers for their alleged lack of critical sense and their blind acceptance of "Christian" premises in their consideration of morality. The work moves into the realm "beyond good and evil" in the sense of leaving behind a traditional morality, which Nietzsche subjects to a destructive critique in favour of what he regards as an affirmative approach that fearlessly confronts the perspectival nature of knowledge and the perilous condition of the modern individual' (based on article in *Ency. Brit.*).

Steiner begins the Preface to the first edition (1895) of *Friedrich Nietzsche Fighter for Freedom*, GA 5 (Spiritual Science Library. Blauvelt, New York 1985): 'When I became acquainted with the works of Friedrich Nietzsche six years ago, ideas had already formed within me which were similar to his. Independently, and from completely different directions, I came to concepts which were in harmony with those Nietzsche expressed in his writings: *Beyond Good and Evil*, *Genealogy of Morals*, and *Twilight of Idols*. In my little book, *The Theory of Knowledge in Goethe's World Conception* (pub. 1886), this same way of implicit thinking is expressed as one find in the works of Nietzsche mentioned above.'

60. A basic account of exercises given by Steiner on bringing rhythm into the breathing and the difference to breathing

exercises as practised in early eastern yoga is to be found in the lecture of 27 May 1922 in GA 212. See also lecture of 30 November 1919 in GA 194; also Hella Wiesberger's detailed commentary 'On the breathing exercises' in GA 267 (not in ET).

61. At the conclusion of the lecture, Oskar Römer expressed his thanks on behalf of all the participants as follows:

'Most highly esteemed Dr Steiner! If today in the name of all the doctors and students here I express our inmost thanks for everything that you have again reported to us of the revelations and stores of wisdom which are a valuable extension, enrichment and—I'd like to say—enlightenment of what you have given us in the previous medical lectures, then this thanks should not only exist in words, which again as sounds will disappear, wafting and dying away, but it shall be thanks expressed in deeds, in deeds where we on the one hand ourselves will work through with greatest diligence and seriousness what you have given us, comparing it with everything that outer science has given us in observable matters. And on the other hand we will carry it out into practical life, letting it flow into what we teach as teachers, letting it flow into our medical practices as doctors. And we can try to make other medical doctors interested in it. For this, though, we need two things. We need firstly the right courage, and secondly the right intelligence, the right tact. We are not to spread out these stores of wisdom without discrimination. We have to be careful, paying attention that what we want to convey to somebody else falls on fruitful ground. These pearls of wisdom we shall not cast before the swine. I would like to say, here we have to be clever like the snakes and without falseness like the doves in representing the truth. We have to be true to ourselves, true towards others, but we also have to be true to Herr Dr Steiner. We have to summon the courage not to be afraid to

appear and not to remain cowardly in silence when Herr Dr
Steiner is being attacked, insulted and jeered. We have to
educate ourselves towards this and develop the strength and
ability in ourselves to bring this amongst people in the correct
professional manner. We have to point out in a right way how
what Herr Dr Steiner gives us is much more splendid and
significant than everything we can gain from the outer
sciences. We must not deny that we are pupils of Herr Dr
Steiner. For this the words Christ spoke to Peter can be a
warning for us, "Before the cock crows you will deny me three
times." We will not deny our master; this we will promise. In
this sense, I thank you, most esteemed Dr Steiner, once again
from all my heart that despite all your other tremendous work
you were prepared to give to us again these treasures of
wisdom.'

Dr. Med. dent Oskar Römer (1866–1952), Professor for
Dental Health, initially in Straßburg, then in Leipzig (1918–
34), where he was Ordinarium (1920), Dekan (1925) and
Rektor (1928). He knew Rudolf Steiner from about 1908.
Member of the Theosophical, later Anthroposophical Society
since 1910. *Published: *Über die Zahnkaries mit Beziehung auf
die Ergebnisse der Geistesforschung Dr. Rudolf Steiners* (Stuttgart
1921).

Lecture 8

62. This refers to the parallel lecture course, held in Dornach 11–
18 April 1921, GA 313.

63. Moritz Benedikt (1835–1920), Austrian physician. With
Cesare Lombroso (1836–1909) he founded a criminal
anthropology. On the alcohol problem, see R. Steiner, *The
Course of My Life*, Chap. 9. Steiner spoke in more detail about
Benedikt in the lecture of 5 November 1921, GA 208. Works
include: *Zur Psychophysik der Moral und des Rechts* (Vienna

1875); *Die Seelenkunde des Menschen als reine Erfahrungs-wissenschaft* (Leipzig 1895); *Das biomechanische (neo-vitalistische) Denken in der Medizin und in der Biologie* (Jena 1893); *Hypnotismus und Suggestion* (Vienna 1894).

64. Details in GA 312, end of lecture 12, also lectures 16 and 17.
65. See lecture of 28 October 1922, in GA 314.
66. See the lectures of 28 and 29 August 1920 in GA 199, the lecture of 22 October 1922 in GA 218, and the answers to questions on 24 April 1924 in GA 316.
67. See the lecture of the same day (28 October 1922) in GA 314.

Note on Rudolf Steiner's Lectures

The lectures and addresses contained in this volume have been translated from the German, which is based on stenographic and other recorded texts that were in most cases never seen or revised by the lecturer. Hence, due to human errors in hearing and transcription, they may contain mistakes and faulty passages. Every effort has been made to ensure that this is not the case. Some of the lectures were given to audiences more familiar with anthroposophy; these are the so-called 'private' or 'members' lectures. Other lectures, like the written works, were intended for the general public. The difference between these, as Rudolf Steiner indicates in his *Autobiography*, is twofold. On the one hand, the members' lectures take for granted a background in and commitment to anthroposophy; in the public lectures this was not the case. At the same time, the members' lectures address the concerns and dilemmas of the members, while the public work arises from, and directly addresses Steiner's own understanding of universal needs. Nevertheless, as Rudolf Steiner stresses: 'Nothing was ever said that was not solely the result of my direct experience of the growing content of anthroposophy. There was never any question of concessions to the prejudices and preferences of the members. Whoever reads these privately printed lectures can take them to represent anthroposophy in the fullest sense. Thus it was possible without hesitation—when the complaints in this direction became too persistent—to depart from the custom of circulating this material "For members only". But it must be borne in mind that faulty passages do occur in these reports not revised by myself.' Earlier in the same chapter, he states: 'Had I been able to correct them [*the private lectures*], the restriction *for members only* would have been unnecessary from the beginning.' The original German editions on which this text is based were published by Rudolf

Steiner Verlag, Dornach, Switzerland in the collected edition (*Gesamtausgabe*, 'GA') of Rudolf Steiner's work. All publications are edited by the Rudolf Steiner Nachlassverwaltung (estate), which wholly owns both Rudolf Steiner Verlag and the Rudolf Steiner Archive.